Topical Issues in Pain 3

T0332209

Physiotherapy Pain Association

Topical Issues in Pain 3

Sympathetic nervous system and pain
Pain management
Clinical effectiveness

Editor
Louis Gifford FCSP BSc MAppSc

Foreword
Vicki Harding MCSP

authorHOUSE®

AuthorHouse™ UK Ltd.
1663 Liberty Drive
Bloomington, IN 47403 USA
www.authorhouse.co.uk
Phone: 0800.197.4150

This book was first published by CNS Press in 2002

Published by AuthorHouse 09/05/2013

ISBN: 978-1-4918-7770-8 (sc)
ISBN: 978-1-4918-7771-5 (hc)
ISBN: 978-1-4918-7772-2 (e)

Foreword

The physiotherapy profession is indeed fortunate to include neuroscientists, therapists with academic and philosophical interests in pain, and clinicians who are neither afraid of using principles and methods developed in other professions to optimise their treatment, nor afraid of working with other professions. This latest volume in the Topical Issues in Pain series reflects a pooling of knowledge from many sources. Within it you will find that members of our profession are also prepared to challenge long-held beliefs, both within and outside the profession. Topical Issues in Pain also allows more extensive reporting of clinical practice, giving insight into the variety of pain management techniques used in more novel and innovative patient-therapist interactions.

The volume opens with Ronald Melzack's historical perspective on his and Pat Wall's work on the gate control theory, and presents his neuromatrix theory: his proposal for the next stage in the evolution of pain concepts. This goes beyond gate control theory in that it addresses how pain is perceived centrally, and makes an important attempt to account for phenomena such as phantom limb pain. It will be fascinating to see when his inclusion of a genetic template within the neuromatrix theory receives backing with scientific data.

Back out in the periphery, the sympathetic nervous system (SNS) has influence over virtually every cell in the body, providing efferent outflow to all the organs and glands, sharing afferent input with the somatic nervous system, having a modulating influence upon the various nerve receptors and muscle spindles, and supporting somatic tissue performance. It is no wonder that the fingerprints of the SNS can be seen all over pain conditions, both acute and chronic, and that certain pain syndromes have features of altered sympathetic activity and pathobiology. Part I enables us to consider the work, knowledge and skills of several of the experts within the profession in relation to the SNS. They encourage us to consider some of the conundrums as well as difficulties that we face with our patients. They also provide suggestions for how we can take our practice forward, with new ideas on how we can approach our patients, guiding them towards understanding, attenuating, and managing their pain.

While the SNS has significant peripheral targets and effects, it also has major influences within the central nervous system. One of these is its close links to emotional states. This has a major impact not only on patients' pain, but also on patient-therapist communication. Part II explores assessment and management of low back pain patients whose distress and anger are significant features of their whole picture.

Clearly, the physiotherapy profession is concerned with pain management, with symptomatic relief, with rehabilitation and with patient education. There is an explosion of new ideas and approaches. Whether we are considering traditional techniques or novel forms of assessment, treatment or patient interaction, clinical effectiveness will be uppermost in our concerns for our patients. Clinical effectiveness based on valid measurement and evidence is a key focus for the PPA, and Part III contributes to its ongoing promotion.

This latest publication from the PPA continues to reflect the work of those speaking at PPA study days and contributing to the PPA programme at the annual CSP Congress. It is an important source for us in these rapidly developing and exciting times!

Vicki Harding
PPA Chairperson
June 2002

Preface

Much of the work of the Physiotherapy Pain Association involves healthy challenges, updates to our knowledge, the improvement of our professional standing in the wider medical community, as well as providing help with the treatment and management of our patients. This third volume of Topical Issues in Pain builds on the previous two and hopefully makes a further contribution to the work and progress already made.

In his book *The Unnatural Nature of Science* Lewis Wolpert challenges what he calls 'common sense' thinking and theories. He argues that common sense reasoning, our 'natural' reasoning, works extremely well for everyday life, but that for science it is quite unsatisfactory. What we naturally think and what may seem quite obvious about a given observation, when probed scientifically, is often found to be quite wrong.

For years physiotherapy models of treatment and reasoning with pain have evolved from just such a 'try it and see,' or 'common sense' linear thinking style and process. If a patient comes in with a leg pain and a therapist tries to help by pressing on the sacroiliac joint for one minute and the patient then moves better, clinical reasoning results in the technique being used again for other similar pains as well as ascribing the cause of the problem to a faulty sacroiliac joint. Occasionally an observation like this may generate a 'new' treatment and assessment paradigm. New therapies, and the hypothetical foundations and rules that are usually generated, often become uncritically established as widely-lionised dogma. Unfortunately, they appear scientific when in fact they are not and those bold enough to criticise them are scolded for undermining the sanctity of the profession's foundations or for making potentially hurtful remarks about the founding godfather figures. Those who move our profession on are important, but the peddling of dogma and unjustified rigid thinking is not good enough any more. Dogma holds back change and it creates a culture whereby those who follow tend to avoid or ignore evidence that conflicts with it. Good science welcomes and thrives on rigorous scrutiny, criticism and collective appraisal. It is time to move on, yet change frustratingly drags its feet.

This book presents the current evidence on what we know about the sympathetic nervous system and the implications it has for patients with complex regional pain syndromes. It also shows us how to understand the evidence based movement and it provides a wealth of clinical material to help us deal with complex pain, complex patients, and complex disability. The material offers understanding, informed opinion and some solutions that may challenge the dogmas we have been taught and which we may still believe. If we are to understand pain and pain related disability better then we need to investigate or side step the old dogma, adjust and accept new scientific rigour, and move on to confront and understand the challenges and changes required.

This comment by Pat Wall, quoted in Chapter 4, nicely sets the scene for the contents of this book: 'It is almost impossible to replace widely accepted medical dogmas, especially where the paradigm being challenged has to be replaced with a more complicated one!' (see page 103.)

Pat Wall died in August 2001. He was a friend of physiotherapy and he particularly respected the Physiotherapy Pain Association for embracing pain science, and its critical yet forward thinking stance. It is especially fitting that this volume opens with an essay by Ronald Melzack, Pat's partner in producing the gate control theory of pain and his close friend.

Thanks to all the authors for their ground-breaking work and for being so patient. Special thanks to my project manager Judy Waters, for organising me and getting the final products so polished, and thanks to my team at home, Philippa and Teresa.

Louis Gifford
July 2002

Contributors

Suzanne Brook MCSP, GradDipPhys
Formerly Clinical Specialist in Pain Management, Physiotherapy
Pain Management Department
The National Hospital for Neurology and Neurosurgery
Queen's Square
London WC1N 3BG UK

Louis Gifford FCSP, BSc, MAppSc
Chartered Physiotherapist
Kestrel, Swanpool
Falmouth, Cornwall TR11 5BD UK

Ralph Hammond MCSP, MSc
Chartered Physiotherapist
Professional Adviser Research and Clinical Effectiveness Unit
Chartered Society of Physiotherapy
14 Bedford Row
London WC1R 4ED UK

Chris Main FBPsS, PhD
Consultant Clinical Psychologist
Department of Behavioural Medicine
Hope Hospital, Salford
Honorary Professor of Behavioural Medicine
University of Manchester
Manchester, UK

Ronald Melzack FRSC, PhD
Professor Emeritus, Department of Psychology
McGill University
Montreal, Canada

Lesley Smith PhD Research Fellow
ICRF/NHS Centre for Statistics in Medicine
Institute of Health Sciences
Old Road, Headington
Oxford OX3 7LF UK

Mick Thacker MCSP, MMACP, GradDipPhys, MSc
Superintendent Physiotherapist
Guy's and St Thomas' NHS Trust
London UK
Research Student, Centre for Neuroscience Research
King's College, London
Lecturer, Physiotherapy Division
King's College, London UK

Paul Watson MCSP, BSc (Hons), MSc, PhD
Consultant AHP and Senior Lecturer in Pain Management and Rehabilitation
Department of Anaesthesia, Pain Management and Critical Care
University of Leicester
Leicester General Hospital
Leicester LE5 UK

Contents

Introductory essay

Gate control theory: on the evolution of pain concepts

Reprinted from Pain Forum: Official Journal of the American Pain Society, Volume 5 pp 128–138, Copyright © 1996 by American Pain Society, with permission from Churchill Livingstone, an imprint of Elsevier Science (USA)

RONALD MELZACK

Theories of pain, like every other kind of theory, evolve in conjunction with the accumulation of scientific facts. Theories give rise to experiments, which generate new facts, and these, in turn, reveal the inadequacies of older theories and provide the foundations for new ones. This article discusses the gate control theory of pain in the perspective of earlier theories and outlines the data that call for a new one. In particular, phantom limb pain cannot be explained by any current theories and reveals that the study of brain function, in general, is in a state of crisis. We have a multitude of facts but no adequate frame-work to incorporate them into a meaningful whole.

A brief history of pain

The theory of pain we inherited in the 20th century was proposed by Descartes three centuries earlier (see Melzack and Wall[32]). Descartes was the first philosopher to be influenced by the scientific method that flourished in the 17th century, and he achieved a major revolution by arguing that the body works like a machine that can be studied by using the experimental methods of physics pioneered by Galileo and others. Although humans, Descartes proposed, have a soul (or mind), the human body is nevertheless, a machine, like an animal's body.

The impact of Descartes' theory was enormous. The history of experiments on the anatomy and physiology of pain during the first half of this century (reviewed in Melzack and Wall[32]) is marked by a search for specific pain fibres and pathways and a pain centre in the brain. The result was a concept

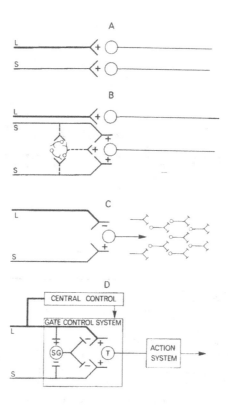

Fig. 1A, B, C, & D Schematic representation of conceptual models of pain mechanisms.

(A) Specificity theory. Large (L) and small (S) fibres are assumed to transmit touch and pain impulses respectively, in separate, specific, straight-through pathways to touch and pain centres in the brain.

(B) Goldscheider's summation theory, showing convergence of small fibres onto a dorsal horn cell. The central network projecting to the central cell represents Livingston's (1943) conceptual model of reverberatory circuits underlying pathological pain states. Touch is assumed to be carried by large fibres.

(C) Sensory interaction theory, in which large (L) fibres inhibit (-) and small (S) fibres excite (+) central transmission neurons. The output projects to spinal cord neurons, which are conceived by Noordenbos (1959) to comprise a multisynaptic afferent system.

(D) Gate control theory. The large (L) and small (S) fibres project to the substantia gelatinosa (SG) and first central transmission (T) cells. The central control trigger is represented by a line running from the large fibre system to central control mechanisms, which in turn project back to the gate control system. The T cells project to the entry cells of the action system. +, excitation; -, inhibition.

From Melzack R 1991 The gate control theory 25 years later: new perspectives on phantom limb pain. In: Bond M, Charlton JE, Woolf CJ (eds) Pain Research and Therapy: Proceedings 6th World Congress on Pain. Elsevier, Amsterdam 9–21 of pain as a specific, straight-through sensory projection system. This rigid anatomy of pain in the 1950s led to attempts to treat severe chronic pain by a variety of neurosurgical lesions. Descartes' specificity theory, then, determined the 'facts' as they were known up to the middle of this century, and even determined therapy.

Specificity theory proposed that injury activates specific pain receptors and fibres that, in turn, project pain impulses through a spinal pain pathway to a pain centre in the brain. The psychological experience of pain, therefore, was virtually equated with peripheral injury. In the 1950s, there was no room for psychological contributions to pain, such as attention, past experience, and the meaning of the situation. Instead, pain experience was held to be proportional to peripheral injury of pathology. Patients who suffered back pain without presenting signs of organic disease were labelled as psychologically disturbed and sent to psychiatrists. The concept, in short, was simple and, not surprisingly, generally failed to help patients who suffered severe chronic pain. To thoughtful clinical observers, specificity theory was clearly wrong.

There were several attempts to find a new theory. The major opponent to specificity was labelled as 'pattern theory', but there were several different pattern theories and they were generally vague and inadequate. However, seen in retrospect, pattern theories gradually evolved and set the stage for the gate control theory (Fig. 1). Goldscheider[5] proposed that central summation in dorsal horns is one of the critical determinants of pain. Livingston's[16] theory postulated a reverberatory circuit in the dorsal horns to explain summation, referred pain, and pain that persisted long after healing was completed. Noordenbos's theory[33] proposed that large-diameter fibres inhibited small-diameter fibres, and he even suggested that the substantia gelatinosa in the dorsal horn plays a major role in the summation and other dynamic processes described by Livingston. However, in none of these theories was there an explicit role for the brain other than as a passive receiver of messages. Nevertheless, the successive theoretical concepts moved the field in the right direction: into the spinal cord and away from the periphery as the exclusive answer to pain.

The evolution of new concepts

Progress in science, according to historians of science such as Thomas Kuhn,[12] occurs in two ways: by the gradual accumulation of information that we call 'facts' and by the rapid jumps in the integration of facts that occur when a new theory, concept, or 'paradigm' is proposed. The former is 'normal science'; the latter is a 'revolution'. The process occurs in a cycle that may involve generations of scientists and take centuries to complete. This historical process is depicted in Figure 2 (see page 4), with specific reference to the history of pain.

The power of theory was summarised briefly by Donald O. Hebb: 'The "realworld" is a construct, and some of the peculiarities of scientific thought become more intelligible when this fact is recognised...Einstein himself in 1926 told Heisenberg it was nonsense to found a theory on observable facts alone: "In reality the very opposite happens. It is theory which decides what we can observe."' (Hebb[7] pp 5–9). In the case of pain, theory not only determines what we observe in physiology, but it determines how we treat people in pain. We now know that neurosurgical lesions to abolish chronic pain usually fail and the pain tends to return. Yet theory and so-called facts about pain fibres and pathways said they should work and neurosurgeons—notwithstanding their own observations on the tendency for pain to return after surgery—continued to carry out cordotomies, rhizotomies, cortical ablations, and so forth. The emphasis was on the temporary successes, not on the long-term follow-up failures.[3,37]

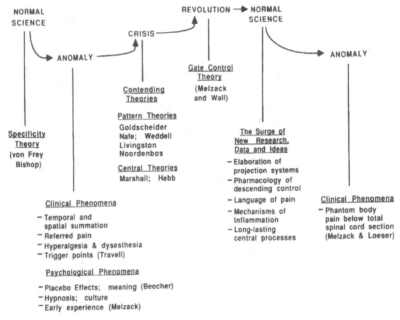

Fig. 2 The pattern of scientific progress according to Kuhn (1970)

'Normal science' is a generally tranquil stage in which scientific data are acquired within the framework of a theory or 'paradigm' that is generally accepted by all or most scientists. During this period, data are obtained that represent an anomaly—they do not fit the accepted paradigm. These data usually lead to several new theories to explain the anomalous data and produce a contentious and unsettled period. Finally, a single theory emerges that becomes the new paradigm and represents a revolution from the old paradigm to the new one. Within this new paradigm, normal science produces new data and proceeds until a period of anomaly again arises, thus leading to a new cycle that culminates in the revolution of a new paradigm. This sequence is shown specifically for pain, with the major events and scientists associated with each stage.

From Melzack R 1991 The gate control theory 25 years later: new perspectives on phantom limb pain. In: Bond M, Charlton JE, Woolf CJ (eds) Pain Research and Therapy: Proceedings 6th world Congress on Pain. Elsevier, Amsterdam 9–21.

Descartes' views have so thoroughly permeated our concepts about physiology and anatomy that we still cannot escape them. In addition to the concept of a specific pain projection system, Descartes left us another legacy that has perverted our understanding of how the nervous system works: it led to psychophysics, the idea that the relationships between sensation and stimulus energy can be expressed in elegant mathematical formulas, suggesting mechanical, immutable laws, like the physics of long ago. Certainly we find these laws—when we use rats and students in artificial laboratory chambers. In the normal world, perception and behaviour are highly variable, with a multitude of contributing factors. Fortunately, psychology has recently undergone major changes.[13] Behaviourism, which ignored the brain and its functions, is vanishing; cognitive psychology, which recognises the variability of perception the malleability of memory, thought, and imagery, has now become the dominant concept.

This new approach in psychology is, happily being paralleled by major changes in our views of brain function. We now know that the brain possesses widely distributed, parallel processing networks and that it produces an excess of neurons and synapses, so that we can conceive of memory as a sculpting process rather than a slow 'cementing' of synapses. This new, dynamic picture of the brain is gradually having an impact on our understanding of pain.

The gate control theory of pain

Science is a highly personal endeavour and it is necessary for me, therefore, to discuss the milieu in which I first approached the problem of pain. The careers of many scientists are launched during the formative years of working on a doctoral thesis, and the concept of 'gating' by the brain evolved during that exciting period of my life. I had the good fortune, in the early 1950s, to have a superb research advisor—Donald O. Hebb—and a challenging problem: pain. Happily, Hebb was then engaged in a long correspondence on the problem of pain with George H. Bishop—a brilliant physiologist who shared Hebb's fascination with the nervous system. Bishop was convinced that pain would one day be explained entirely (or primarily) in terms of the sizes of fibres (which his research helped to sort out) and their projections to the brain. However, the brief section on pain in Hebb's book[7] *The Organisation of Behaviour*, which ascribed pain to abnormal patterns of firing in the brain, intrigued Bishop. In the course of the exchange of ideas, Hebb described his ongoing research on the role of early sensory experience on adult behaviour in Scottish terriers and stated his hope that experiments such as these might throw light on the role of learning in pain perception.

Here, suddenly, a possible PhD thesis topic leaped out at me. Scottish terriers were already being raised in social isolation in Hebb's laboratory in special sensory-restriction cages (kennel cages with boards on the side and top), and littermate controls were being raised in homes as pets. Hebb was interested in the effects of sensory-social restriction on intelligence. I was now curious to know whether this kind of restriction had an effect on pain perception.

When the restricted dogs were removed from their cages, they became extremely excited. They ran wildly around the laboratory rooms, in sharp contrast to the controls who cautiously explored every important place and object. At a suitable time, I lit a match in the presence of a restricted dog. He sniffed it, withdrew reflexively for a moment and sniffed again—and again and again. The other restricted dogs behaved essentially the same way. The control dogs, in sharp contrast, carefully avoided the flaming match so that I had to chase after them. The few that ventured one sniff would not try another. Similar behaviour was observed when the stimulus was pricking the skin was a dissecting needle.

More litters of dogs and more elegant testing sessions led to similar observations.[27] The question raised by these observations was this: Did the dogs really not feel pain or did they have to learn the meaning of different stimuli until they learned that flaming matches or sharp needles were different and more dangerous than other kinds of inputs? Several years of research subsequently led me to conclude that the restricted dogs had difficulty in discriminating among stimuli, largely because of their high level of arousal.[18] I developed the hypothesis that part of the input from an object such as a flaming match must travel rapidly up the largest fibres and fastest pathways to the brain and activate neural processes that act down on the more slowly conducted input. The information descending from the brain, I proposed, acted at levels that had to be below the brainstem reticular formation. The brains of restricted dogs, without the advantage of prior learning, allowed all information to ascend to the brain. Flaming matches and dissecting needles were no more important than anything else in the environment, and the massive, unfiltered sensory input produced high levels of reticular arousal. The restricted dogs, I believed, could indeed feel pain, but the irrelevant messages were not being inhibited below the level of the reticular formation, and the relevant injury signals failed to rise above the background noise.

In 1959, then, when I was appointed assistant professor of psychology at Massachusetts Institute of Technology and met a young professor of biology, Patrick Wall, we both had ideas that we shared: pain is due to patterns of nerve impulses rather than straight-line transmission of modality-specific impulses to a pain centre; information that arrives at the spinal cord is filtered and selected on the basis of the total pattern of activity in stimulated fibres as well as by descending information from the brain. Wall and I wrote a paper on somesthesis that was published in *Brain* in 1962,[30] and we then decided to write a paper specifically on pain, which was published in *Science* in 1965.[31] The development of the gate control theory has been described elsewhere.[22] The final model is shown in Figure 1 in the context of earlier theories of pain, It is evident that it is the first theory of pain that incorporated the central control processes of the brain.

The gate control theory of pain (Fig. 1D) is based on the following propositions:

- The transmission of nerve impulses from afferent fibres to spinal cord transmission (T) cells is modulated by a spinal gating mechanism in the dorsal horn.
- The spinal gating mechanism is influenced by the relative amount of activity in large-diameter (L) and small-diameter (S) fibres: activity in large fibres tends to inhibit transmission (close the gate) while small-fibre activity tends to facilitate transmission (open the gate).
- The spinal gating mechanism is influenced by nerve impulses that descend from the brain.
- A specialised system of large-diameter, rapidly conducting fibres (the central control trigger) activates selective cognitive processes that then influence, by way of descending fibres, the modulating properties of the spinal gating mechanism.
- When the output of the spinal cord transmission (T) cells exceeds a critical level, it activates the action system—those neural areas that underlie the complex, sequential patterns of behaviour and experience characteristic of pain.

When the gate control theory was published, Wall and I were astonished by the reception. The theory generated vigorous (sometimes vicious) debate, as well as a great deal of research to disprove or support the theory. The search for specific pain fibres and spinal cells by our opponents now became almost frantic. It was not until the mid-1970s that the gate control theory was presented in almost every major textbook in the biological and medical sciences. At the same time there was an explosion in research on the physiology and pharmacology of the dorsal horns and the descending control systems.

The theory's emphasis on the modulation of inputs in the spinal dorsal horns and the dynamic role of the brain in pain processes had a clinical as well as a scientific impact. Psychological factors, which were previously dismissed as 'reactions to pain', were now seen to be an integral part of pain processing and new avenues for pain control were opened. Similarly, cutting nerves and pathways was gradually replaced by a host of methods to modulate the input. Physical therapists and other health care professionals who use a multitude of modulation techniques were brought into the picture, and transcutaneous electrical nerve stimulation became an important modality for the treatment of chronic and acute pain. The current status of pain research and therapy has been evaluated[32] and indicates that, despite the addition of a massive amount of detail, the conceptual components of the theory remain basically intact after more than 30 years.

Beyond the gate

I believe the great challenge ahead of us is to understand brain function. Kenneth Casey and I[25] made a start by trying to convince our colleagues that specialised systems in the brain are involved in the sensory-discriminative, motivational-affective, and evaluative dimensions of pain (Fig. 3). These phrases seemed strange when we coined them, but they are now used so frequently and seem so 'logical' that they have become part of our language. So too, the McGill Pain Questionnaire, which taps into subjective experience—one of the functions of the brain—is widely used to measure pain.[19,29] Later articles tried to understand the spinal and cerebral systems that underlie acute and chronic pain,[2] and we have gained a far better understanding of the analgesic effects of morphine.[21,39]

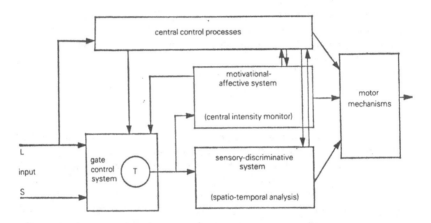

Fig. 3 Conceptual model of the sensory, motivational, and central control determinants of pain. The output of the T (transmission) cells of the gate control system projects to the sensory-discriminative system and the motivational-affective system. The central control trigger is represented by a line running from the large fibre system to central control processes; these, in turn, project back to the gate control system, and to the sensory-discriminative and motivational-affective systems. All three systems interact with one another, and project to the motor system.

From Melzack R, Casey K 1968 Sensory, motivational and central control determinants of pain; a new conceptual model. In: Kenshalo D (ed) The Skin Senses. Charles C. Thomas, Springfield, IL 423–443

The gate control theory had another, unexpected effect. The increasing visits to China by Westerners, beginning in the early 1970s, led to a fascination with acupuncture. Interestingly, the explanation for the ability of acupuncture to relieve some kinds of pain, given by Chinese scientists with a 'Western' training and orientation, was the gate control theory. Acupuncture needles were assumed to activate large fibres that closed the gate to inputs from slowly conducting 'pain fibres.' This explanation lent credibility to acupuncture for pain, and a surge of research on the topic occurred in Western laboratories of physiology, psychology, and pharmacology.[24]

An early study I carried out with W. K. Livingston during three postdoctoral years in his laboratory led to the discovery that the area surrounding the aqueduct in the midbrain exerted a tonic inhibitory effect on pain.[28] This experiment was, in large part, the basis for postulating a descending inhibitory control in the gate theory. It also led directly to Reynolds' demonstration[24] that electrical stimulation of the periaqueductal gray produced analgesia. This study was followed by Liebeskind and Paul's[15] research on the mechanisms of the descending inhibition and by the discovery of pharmacological substances such as endorphins that contribute to it.[4] My interest in the observation that 'pain takes away pain', in which I postulated that descending inhibition tends to be activated by intense inputs, led a series of studies on intense transcutaneous electrical nerve stimulation.[20] Later, a series of definitive studies on 'diffuse noxious inhibitory controls' was carried out by Besson and colleagues,[14] which firmly established the power of descending inhibitory controls.

In 1978, John Loeser and I[26] described severe pains in the phantom body of paraplegics with verified total sections of the spinal cord and proposed a central 'pattern generating mechanism' above the level of the section (Fig. 4). This concept represented a major advance: it did not merely extend the gate, it said that pain could be generated by brain mechanisms in paraplegics in the absence of a spinal gate because the brain is completely disconnected from the cord. Psychophysical specificity, in such a concept, makes no sense and we must explore how patterns of nerve impulses generated in the brain can give rise to somesthetic experience. This concept does not diminish the role of sensory inputs and spinal processing in pain due to injury, inflammation, and other pathology. It simply provides a new perspective in which the brain synthesises raw sensory inputs and generates perceptual experience. This approach seems radical and difficult to comprehend, but I am convinced that it is the logical extension of concepts that began with the gate control theory's incorporation of the brain in the attempt to understand pain.

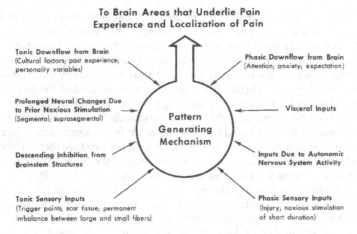

Fig. 4 Concept of a pattern generating mechanism controlled by multiple inputs

From Melzack R, Loeser JD 1978 Phantom body pain in paraplegics: evidence for a central 'pattern generating mechanism' for pain. Pain 4:195–210

Phantom limbs and the concept of a neuromatrix

It is evident that the gate control theory has taken us a long way. Yet, as historians of science have pointed out, good theories are instrumental in producing facts that eventually require a new theory to incorporate them. And this is what has happened. It is possible to make adjustments to the gate theory so that, for example, it includes long-lasting activity of the sort Wall[41] has described. But there is a set of observations on pain in paraplegics that just does not fit the theory. This does not negate the gate theory, of course. Peripheral and spinal processes are obviously an important part of pain, and we need to know more about the mechanisms of peripheral inflammation, spinal modulation, midbrain descending control, and so forth. But the data on painful phantoms below the level of total spinal section[26] indicate that we need to go beyond the foramen magnum and into the brain.[22,23]

Now let me make it clear that I mean more than just the spinal projection systems to thalamus and cortex. These are important, of course, but they mark just the beginning of the psychological process that underlies perception. The cortex, White and Sweet[44] have made amply clear, is not the pain centre and neither is the thalamus.[37] The areas of the brain involved in pain experience and behaviour are very extensive. They must include somatosensory projections as well as the limbic system. Furthermore, because our body perceptions include visual and vestibular mechanisms as well as cognitive processes, widespread areas of the brain must be involved in pain. Yet the plain fact is that we do not have an adequate theory of how the brain works.

My analysis of phantom limb phenomena[22,23] has led to four conclusions that point to a new conceptual nervous system. First, because the phantom limb (or other body part) feels so real, it is reasonable to conclude that the body we normally feel is subserved by the same neural processes in the brain; these brain processes are normally activated and modulated by inputs from the body, but they can act in the absence of any inputs. Second, all the qualities we normally feel from the body, including pain, are also felt in the absence of inputs from the body; from this we may conclude that the origins of the patterns that underlie the qualities of experience lie in neural networks in the brain; stimuli may trigger the patterns but do not produce them. Third, the body is perceived as a unity and is identified as the 'self' distinct from other people and the surrounding world. The experience of a unity of such diverse feelings, including the self as the point of orientation in the surrounding environment, is produced by central neural processes and cannot derive from the peripheral nervous system or spinal cord. Fourth, the brain processes that underlie the body self are, to an important extent that can no longer be ignored, 'built-in' by genetic specification, although this built-in substrate must, of course, be modified by experience. These conclusions provide the basis of the new conceptual model.

Outline of the theory

The anatomical substrate of the body-self, I propose, is a large, widespread network of neurons that consists of loops between the thalamus and cortex as well as between the cortex and limbic system. I have labelled the entire network, whose spatial distribution and synaptic links are initially determined genetically and are later sculpted by sensory inputs, as a *neuromatrix*. The loops diverge to permit parallel processing in different components of the neuromatrix and converge repeatedly to permit interactions between the output products of processing. The repeated cyclical processing and synthesis of nerve impulses through the neuromatrix imparts a characteristic pattern: the *neurosignature*. The neurosignature of the neuromatrix is imparted on all nerve impulse patterns that flow through it; the neurosignature is produced by the patterns of synaptic connections in the entire neuromatrix. All inputs from the body undergo cyclical processing and synthesis so that characteristic patterns are impressed on them in the neuromatrix. Portions of the neuromatrix are specialized to process information related to major sensory events (such as injury, temperature change, and stimulation of erogenous tissue) and may be labelled as neuromodules, which impress subsignatures on the larger neurosignature.

The neurosignature, which is a continuous outflow from the body-self neuromatrix, is projected to areas in the brain—the *sentient neural hub*—in which the stream of nerve impulses (the neurosignature modulated by ongoing inputs) is converted into a continually changing stream of awareness. Furthermore, the neurosignature patterns may also activate a neuromatrix to produce movement. That is, the signature patterns bifurcate so that a pattern proceeds to the sentient neural hub (where the pattern is converted into the experience of movement), and a similar pattern proceeds through a neuromatrix that eventually activates spinal cord neurons to produce muscle patterns for complex actions.

The four components of the new conceptual nervous system, then, are (1) the body-self neuromatrix; (2) cyclical processing and sysnthesis, in which the neurosignature is produced; (3) the sentient neural hub, which converts (transduces) the flow of neurosignatures into the flow of awareness; and (4) activation of an action neuromatrix to provide the pattern of movements to bring about the desired goal.

The body-self neuromatrix

The body is felt as a unity, with different qualities at different times and I believe, the brain mechanism that underlies the experience also comprises a unified system that acts as a whole and produces a neurosignature pattern of a whole body. The conceptualisation of this unified brain mechanism lies at the heart of the new theory and I believe the word 'neuromatrix' best characterises it. 'Matrix' has several definitions in Webster's dictionary,[43] and some of them imply precisely the properties of the neuromatrix as I conceive of it. First, a matrix is defined as 'something within which something else originates, takes from or develops'. This is exactly what I wish to imply: the neuromatrix (not the stimulus, peripheral nerves, or 'brain centre') is the origin of the neurosignature; the neurosignature originates and takes form in the neuromatrix. Though the neurosignature may be triggered or modulated by input, the input is only a 'trigger' and does not produce the neurosignature itself. Matrix is also defined as a 'mold' or 'die' that leaves an imprint on something else. In this sense, the neuromatrix 'casts' its distinctive signature on all inputs (nerve impulse patterns) that flow through it. Finally, matrix is defined as 'an array of circuit elements…for performing a specific function as interconnected'. The array of neurons in a neuromatrix, I propose, is genetically programmed to perform the specific function of producing the signature pattern. The final, integrated neurosignature pattern for the body self ultimately produces awareness and action.

For these reasons, the term neuromatrix seems to be appropriate. The neuromatrix, distributed throughout many areas of the brain, comprises a widespread network of neurons that generates patterns, processes information that flows through it, and ultimately produces the pattern that is felt as a whole body. The stream of neurosignature output with constantly varying patterns riding on the main signature pattern produces the feelings of the whole body with constantly changing qualities.

Psychological reasons for a neuromatrix

It is incomprehensible to me how individual bits of information from skin, joints, or muscles can all come together to produce the experience of a coherent, articulated body. At any instant in time, millions of nerve impulses arrive at the brain from all the body's sensory systems, including the proprioceptive and vestibular systems. How can all this be integrated in a constantly changing unity of experience? Where does it all come together?

I cannot imagine how all these bits are added up to produce a whole. But I can visualise a genetically built-in neuromatrix for the whole body, producing a characteristic neurosignature for the body that carries with it patterns for the myriad qualities we feel. The neuromatrix, as I conceive of it, produces a continuous message that represents the whole body in which details are differentiated within the whole as inputs come into it. We start from the top, with the experience of a unity of the body, and look for differentiation of detail within the whole. The neuromatrix, then, is a template of the whole, which provides the characteristic neural pattern for the whole body (the body's neurosignature), as well as subsets of signature patterns (from neuromodules) that relate to events at (or in) different parts of the body.

These views are in sharp contrast to the classical specificity theory, in which the qualities of experience are presumed to be inherent in peripheral nerve fibres. Pain is not injury; the quality of pain experiences must not be confused with the physical event of breaking skin or bone. Warmth and cold are not 'out there" temperature changes occur 'out there' but the qualities of experience must be generated by structures in the brain. There are no external equivalents to stinging, smarting, tickling, itch; the qualities are produced by built-in neuromodules whose neurosignatures innately produce the qualities.

We do not learn to feel qualities of experience; our brains are built to produce them. The inadequacy of the traditional peripheralist view becomes especially evident when we consider paraplegics with high-level complete spinal breaks. In spite of the absence of inputs from the body, virtually every quality of sensation and affect is experienced. It is known that the absence of input produces hyperactivity and abnormal firing patterns in spinal cells above the level of the break.[26] But how, from this jumble of activity, do we get the meaningful experience of movement, the co-ordination of limbs with other limbs, cramping pain in specific (non-existent) muscle groups, and so on? This must occur in the brain, in which neurosignatures are produced by neuromatrixes that are triggered by the output of hyperactive cells.

When all sensory systems are intact, inputs modulate the continuous neuromatrix output to produce the wide variety of experiences we feel. We may feel position, warmth, and several kinds of pain and pressure all at once. It is a single unitary feeling, just as an orchestra produces a single unitary sound at any moment even though the sound comprises violins, cellos, horns and so forth. Similarly, at a particular moment in time, we feel complex qualities from all of the body. In addition, our experience of the body includes visual images, affect, 'knowledge' of the self (versus not-self), as well as the meaning of body parts in terms of social norms and values. I cannot conceive of all of these bits and pieces coming together to produce a unitary body-self, but I can visualise a neuromatrix that impresses a characteristic signature on all the inputs that converge on it and thereby produces the never ending stream of feeling from the body.

The experience of the body-self involves multiple dimensions—sensory, affective, evaluative, postural, and many others. The sensory dimensions are subserved, in part at least, by portions of the neuromatrix that lie in the sensory projection areas of the brain; the affective dimensions, I assume, are subserved by areas in the brainstem and limbic system. Each major psychological dimension (or quality) of experience, I propose, is subserved by a particular portion of the neuromatrix that contributes a distinct portion of the total neurosignature. To use a musical analogy once again, it is like the strings, tympani, woodwinds, and brasses of a symphony orchestra, which each comprise a part of the whole; each makes its unique contribution yet is an integral part of a single symphony that varies continually from beginning to end.

The neuromatrix resembles Hebb's 'cell assembly' by being a widespread network of cells that subserves a particular psychological function. However, Hebb[7] conceived of the cell assembly as a network developed by gradual sensory learning, while I, instead, propose that the structure of the neuromatrix is predominantly determined by genetic factors, although its eventual synaptic architecture is influenced by sensory inputs. This emphasis on the genetic contribution to the brain does not diminish the importance of sensory inputs. The neuromatrix is a psychologically meaningful unit, developed by both heredity and learning, that represents an entire unified entity.

Action patterns: the action neuromatrix

The output of the body neuromatrix, I have proposed above, is directed at two systems; the neuromatrix that produces awareness of the output and a neuromatrix involved in overt action patterns. In this discussion, it is important to keep in mind that, just as there is a steady stream of awareness, there is also a steady output of behaviour (including movements during sleep).

It is important to recognise that behaviour occurs only after the input has been, at least partially, synthesised and recognised. For example, when we respond to the experience of pain or itch, it is evident that the experience has been synthesised by the body-self neuromatrix (or relevant neuromodules) sufficiently for the neuromatrix to have imparted the neurosignature patterns that underlie the quality of experience, affect, and meaning. Apart from a few reflexes (such as withdrawal of a limb, eye-blink, and so on), behaviour occurs only after inputs have been analysed and synthesised sufficiently to produce meaningful experience. When we reach for an apple, the visual input has clearly been synthesised by a neuromatrix so that it has three-dimensional shape, colour, and meaning as an edible, desirable object, all of which are produced by the brain and are not in the object 'out there'. When we respond to pain (by withdrawal or even by telephoning for an ambulance), we respond to an experience that has sensory qualities, affect, and meaning as a dangerous (or potentially dangerous) event to the body.

I propose that after inputs from the body undergo transformation in the body-neuromatrix, the appropriate action patterns are activated concurrently (or nearly so) with the neuromatrix for experience. Thus, in the action-neuromatrix, cyclical processing and synthesis produces activation of several possible patterns and their successive elimination until one particular pattern emerges as the most appropriate for the circumstances at the moment. In this way, input and output are synthesised simultaneously, in parallel, not in series. This permits a smooth, continuous stream of action patterns.

The command, which originates in the brain, to perform a pattern such as running activates the neuromodule, which then produces firing in sequences of neurons that send precise messages through ventral horn neuron pools to appropriate sets of muscles. At the same time the output patterns from the body-neuromatrix that engage the neuromodules for particular actions are also projected to the sentient neural hub and produce experience. In this way, the brain commands may produce the experience of movement of phantom limbs even though there are no limbs to move and no proprioceptive feed-back. Indeed, reports by paraplegics of terrible fatigue as a result of persistent bicycling movements (like the painful fatigue in a tightly clenched phantom fist in arm amputees) indicate that feelings of effort and fatigue are produced by the signature of a neuromodule rather than particular input patterns from muscles and joints.

Implications of the new concept

Phantom limb pain

The new theory of brain function, proposed on the basis of phantom limb phenomena, provides an explanation for phantom limb pain. Amputees suffer burning, cramping and other qualities of pain. An excellent series of studies[8,11] found that 72% of amputees had phantom limb pain a week after amputation and that 60% had pain six months later. Even seven years after amputation 60% still continued to suffer phantom limb pain, which means that only about 10% to 12% of amputees obtain pain relief. The pain is remarkably intractable; although many forms of treatment have been tried, none has proved to be particularly efficacious.[36]

Why is there so much pain in phantom limbs? I believe that the active body-neuromatrix, in the absence of modulating inputs from the limbs or body, produces a neurosignature pattern, including the high-frequency, bursting pattern that typically follows deafferentation, which is transduced in the sentient neural hub into a hot or burning quality. The cramping pain, however, may be due to messages from the action-neuromodule to move muscles in order to produce movement. In the absence of the limbs, the messages to move the muscles become more frequent and 'stronger' in the attempt to move the limb. The end result of the output message may be felt as cramping muscle pain. Shooting pains may have a similar origin, in which action-neuromodules attempt to move the body and send out abnormal patterns that are felt as shooting pain. The origins of these pains, then, lie in the brain.

Recent research

Surgical removal of the somatosensory areas of the cortex or thalamus fails to relieve phantom limb pain.[44] However, the new theory conceives of a neuromatrix that extends throughout selective areas of the whole brain. Thus, to destroy the neuromatrix for the body-self, which generates the neurosignature pattern for pain, is impossible. However, if the neurosignature for pain is generated by cyclical processing and synthesis, then it may be possible to block it by injecting a local anaesthetic into a discrete area. Such an injection would be relatively easy and harmless to carry out and could bring relief that extends beyond the duration of the anaesthetic.

In the first study on this problem, Tasker and I[38] injected the local anaesthetic lidocaine into the lateral hypothalamus—an area we considered to be strategic for a neuromatrix for the body-self and pain. We found that freely moving rats that received the injection showed a significant reduction of pain in the formalin test, which produces a moderately intense pain for 1 to 2 hours and has many of the characteristics of injury-produced pain in humans. However, the injection had no effect on tail-flick pain, which is primarily a spinally mediated reflex. Moreover, lidocaine injected into adjacent hypothalamic structures (including the medial hypothalamus) had no effect on the formalin-test pain, indicating that the analgesia was produced by local anaesthesia of a specific group of neurons. Since the analgesia was bilateral, it is reasonable to assume that the lateral hypothalamus contains neurons that are important for producing the neurosignature for in both sides of the body.

Recently, Vaccarino and I[40] injected lidocaine into the cingulum bundle and other areas that seem to be strategically located in the neuromatrix for the synthesis of the neurosignature for pain. The results showed that the lidocaine produces striking decreases in pain in the formalin test, as well as in self-mutilation produced by pain or dysesthesia after peripheral nerve lesions. McKenna and I[17] obtained similar results after injection of lidocaine into the dentate nucleus. These exciting results suggest a valuable new approach for the study of pain. If, ultimately, they lead to the relief of pain and suffering, the neuromatrix theory will have served at least one valuable function.

My students and I have also gathered some direct evidence supporting my suggestion that the brain—and, by implication, the neuromatrix—can generate sensation on its own. The formalin pain test produces an 'early' pain that rapidly rises and falls in intensity during the first 5 minutes after the injection, followed by a 'late' pain, which begins about 15 minutes after the injections and persists for about an hour. By means of this test, Coderre, Vaccarino and I[1] found that an anaesthetic block of the paw completely obliterates the late pain, but only if the anaesthetic is delivered in time to prevent the early response. Once the early pain occurs, the drug only partly reduces the later response. This observation of pain continuing even after the nerves carrying pain signals are blocked implies that long-lasting pain (such as that in phantoms) is determined not only by sensory stimulation during the discomfort but also by brain processes that persist without continual priming.

In a related study, Katz et al[10] showed that an injury of a rat's paw before it is totally denervated leaves a lasting memory that influences rat's later perception of pain in the 'phantom' of the denervated paw. These 'pain memories' are consistent with earlier observations that the pain felt in phantom limbs in humans often resembles the pains of earlier injuries of the limbs prior to amputation.[9]

The phenomenon of phantom limbs has allowed me to examine some fundamental assumptions in psychology. One assumption is that sensations are produced only by stimuli and that perceptions in the absence of stimuli are psychologically abnormal. Yet phantom limbs, as well as phantom seeing,[35] indicate this notion is wrong. The brain does more than detect and analyse inputs; it generates perceptual experience even when no external inputs occur.

Another entrenched assumption is that perception of one's body results from sensory inputs that leave a memory in the brain; the total of theses signals becomes the body image. But the existence of phantoms in people born without a limb or who have lost a limb at an early age suggests that the neural networks for perceiving the body and its parts are built into the brain. The absence of inputs does not stop the networks from generating messages about missing body parts; they continue to produce such messages throughout life. In short, phantom limbs are a mystery only if we assume the body sends sensory messages to a passively receiving brain. Phantoms become comprehensible once we recognise that the brain generates the experience of the body. Sensory inputs merely modulate that experience; they do not directly cause it.

REFERENCES

1   Coderre TJ, Vaccarino AL, Melzack R 1990 Central nervous system plasticity in the tonic pain response to subcutaneous formalin injection. Brain Research 535:155–158
2   Dennis SG, Melzack R 1977 Pain-signalling systems in the dorsal and ventral spinal cord. Pain 4:97–132
3   Drake CG, McKenzie KG 1953 Mesencephalic tractotomy for pain. Journal of Neurosurgery 10:457–462
4   Fields HL, Basbaum AL 1994 Central nervous system mechanisms of pain modulation In: Wall PD, Melzack R (eds) Textbook of Pain 3rd edn. Churchill Livingstone, Edinburgh 243–257
5   Goldscheider A 1894 Uber den Schmerzs in Pysiologischer und klinischer Hinsicht. Hirschwald, Berlin
6   Hebb DO 1975 Science and the world of imagination. Canadian Psychology 16:4–11
7   Hebb DO 1949 The Organisation of Behaviour. Wiley, New York
8   Jensen TS, Krebs B, Nielson J, Rasmussen P 1985 Immediate and long-term phantom limb pain in amputees: Incidence, clinical characteristics and relationship to preamputation limb pain. Pain 21:267–278
9   Katz J, Melzack R 1990 Pain 'memories' in phantom limbs: Review and clinical observation. Pain 43: 319–336
10 Katz J, Vaccarino AL, Coderre TJ, Melzack R 1991 Injury prior to neurectomy alters the pattern of autotomy in rats. Anesthesiology 75:876–883
11 Krebs B, Jensen S, Kroner K, Nielsen J, Jorgenssen HS 1984 Phantom limb phenomena in amputees 7 years after limb amputation. Pain Supplement 2:S85
12 Kuhn TS 1970 The Structure of Scientific Revolutions 2rd edn. University of Chicago Press, Chicago
13 Leahey TH 1980 A History of Psychology. Prentice Hall, Englewood Cliffs, NJ
14 Le Bars D, Dickenson AH, Besson JM 1983 Opiate analgesia and descending control systems. In: Bonical JJ, Lindblom U, Iggo A (eds) Advances in Pain Research and Therapy: Proceedings 3rd World Congress on Pain Vol. 5. Raven Press, New York 341–372
15 Liebeskind JC, Paul LA 1977 Psychological and physiological mechanisms of pain. Annual Review of Psychology 28:41–60
16 Livingston WK 1943 Pain Mechanisms. Macmillan, New York
17 McKenna JE, Melzack R 1992 Analgesia produced by lidocaine microinjection into the dentate gyrus. Pain 49:105–112
18 Melzack R 1965 Effects of early experience on behaviour: experimental and conceptual considerations. In: Hoch P, Zubin J (eds) Psychopathology of Perception. Grune & Stratton, New York 271–299

19 Melzack R 1975 The McGill pain questionnaire: major properties and scoring methods. Pain 1:277–299
20 Melzack R 1975 Prolonged relief of pain by brief, intense transcutaneous somatic stimulation. Pain 1:357–373
21 Melzack R 1988 The tragedy of needless pain: a call for social action. In: Dubner R, Gebhart GF, Bond MR (eds) Proceedings 5th World Congress on Pain. Elsevier, Amsterdam, 1–11
22 Melzack R 1989 Phantom limbs, the self and the brain (The D.O. Hebb Memorial Lecture) Canadian Psychology 30:1–14
23 Melzack R 1991 The gate control theory 25 years later: new perspectives on phantom limb pain.. In: Bond M, Charlton J E, Woolf CJ (eds) Pain Research and Therapy: Proceedings 6th World Congress on Pain. Elsevier, Amsterdam 9–21
24 Melzack R 1994 Folk medicine and the sensory modulation of pain. In: Wall PD, Melzack R (eds) Textbook of pain 3rd edn. Churchill Livngstone, Edinburgh 1209–1217
25 Melzack R, Casey KL 1968 Sensory, motivational and central control determinants of pain: a new conceptual model. In: Kenshalo D (ed) The Skin Senses. Charles C. Thomas, Springfield, IL 423–443
26 Melzack R, Loeser JD 1978 Phantom body pain in paraplegics: evidence for a central 'pattern generating mechanism' for pain. Pain 4:195–210
27 Melzack R, Scott TH 1957 The effects of early experience on the response to pain. Journal of Comparative Physiology and Pyschology 50:155–161
28 Melzack R, Stotler WA, Livingston WK 1958 Effects of discrete brainstem lesions in cats on perception of noxious stimulation. Journal of Neurophysiology 21:353–367
29 Melzack R, Torgerson WR 1971 The language of pain. Anesthesiology 34:50–59
30 Melzack R, Wall PD 1962 On the nature of cutaneous sensory mechanisms. Brain 85:331–356
31 Melzack R, Wall PD 1965 Pain mechanisms: a new theory. Science 150:971–979
32 Melzack R, Wall PD 1988 The challenge of pain 2nd edn. Penguin Books, London
33 Noordenbos W 1959 Pain. Elsevier, Amsterdam
34 Reynolds DV 1969 Surgery in the rat during electrical analgesia induced by focal brain stimulation. Science 164:444–445
35 Schultz G, Melzack R 1991 The Charles Bonnet syndrome: 'phantom visual images.' Perception 20:809–825
36 Sherman RA, Sherman CJ, Gall NG 1980 A survey of current phantom limb pain treatment in the United States. Pain 8:85–90
37 Speigel EA, Wycis HT 1966 Present status of stereoencephalotomies for pain relief. Conf Neurol 27:7–17
38 Tasker RAR, Choiniere M, Libman SM., Melzack R 1987 Analgesia produced by injection of lidocaine into the lateral hypothalamus. Pain 31:237–248
39 Twycross RG 1994 Opioids. In: Wall PD, Melzack R (eds) Textbook of Pain 3rd edn. Churchill Livingstone, Edinburgh 943–962
40 Vaccarino AL, Melzack R 1992 Temporal processes of formalin pain: differential role of the cingulum bundle, fornix pathway and medial bulboreticular formation. Pain 49:257–271
41 Wall PD 1989 Introduction. In: Wall PD, Melzack R (eds) Textbook of Pain 2nd edn. Churchill Livingstone, Edinburgh 1–18
42 Wall PD, Melzack R (eds) 1994 Textbook of Pain 3rd edn. Churchill Livingstone, Edinburgh
43 Webster's Seventh New Collegiate Dictionary 1967 Merriam Co, Springfield, MA, 522
44 White JC, Sweet WH 1969 Pain and the Neurosurgeon. Charles C. Thomas, Springfield, IL

1

Sympathetic nervous system and pain

1

A clinical overview of the autonomic nervous system, the supply to the gut and mind–body pathways

LOUIS GIFFORD AND MICK THACKER

Introduction

The autonomic nervous system (ANS) is an 'output', 'effector' or 'motor' system (see Gifford 1998b)—i.e. it responds to the demands of the sensory systems and the central nervous system (CNS) by producing an effect on the tissues it supplies. There are no sympathetic or parasympathetic sensory (afferent) fibres as such, although a great many visceral sensory fibres do travel in nerves like the vagus and splanchnic, which are commonly described in parasympathetic and sympathetic sections of anatomy texts and often referred to as 'sympathetic afferents' (see discussion of visceral afferents below).

Since the ANS is an output system, its role in pain states has to be secondary to its effects on sensory systems (see following chapters).

ANS fibres create their 'effects' via electrochemical stimulation of smooth muscles or glands. Their secretions also produce direct chemical effects on the tissues they innervate and thus change their chemical characteristics. Any chemical or physiological tissue changes may in turn be fed back to the CNS via stimulation of sensory afferent pathways. This is important because ANS activity has been implicated not only in producing and modulating nociception and pain, but also as playing a role in the expression and conscious awareness of emotions (see Meyers 1986). Recent studies show, for example, that different emotions (anger, fear, disgust, sadness, happiness, surprise) can be distinguished to some extent on the basis of different autonomic nervous system responses (like skin temperature and heart rate) (LeDoux 1998, p 292). We all know that strong emotions are expressed as bodily sensations and that 'gut feelings' play crucial roles in our emotional experiences and can have a strong impact on our decision making processes (Damasio 1995, LeDoux 1998, Damasio 2000).

In their detailed overview of the ANS, Janig and Habler (1999) go out of their way to debunk the traditional descriptions of the ANS and the view that it is 'all or nothing' and general in its mode of action. In parallel with the neuroendocrine system, the ANS regulates target organs in order to maintain the homeostasis of the body. Simply, it adapts, adjusts and co-ordinates appropriate systems so as to produce the required physiological conditions for life, which includes, any required physical activity. In this way it is involved in producing and co-ordinating the necessary physiological responses for activities like moving, resting, sleeping, feeding and digestion, sex, pregnancy and nurturing, growth and repair and all extreme responses relating to threatening and stressful situations. This includes responding to tissue injury and to pain.

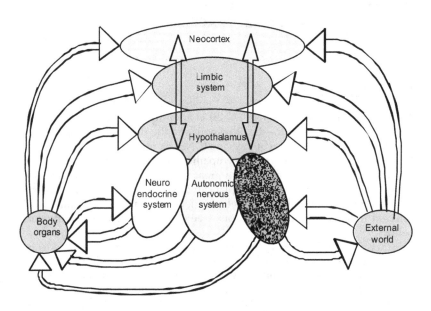

Fig. 1.1 A modified version of Janig and Habler's model of the integration and relationships of the brain and body. What it so nicely illustrates are the forward and back communication links between all levels of the nervous system, the body, and the environment. Communication is via neuronal, hormonal and humoral pathways.

Adapted from: Janig W, Habler HJ 1999 Organization of the autonomic nervous system: structure and function. In: Appenzeller O (ed) Handbook of Clinical Neurology Vol 74 (30): The Autonomic Nervous System Part 1: Normal Functions. Elsevier, Amsterdam

ANS activities can be viewed as being governed by the commands it receives from the modules of the CNS that 'scrutinise and appraise' the sensory and incoming information received (Gifford 1998). Thus, environmental inputs from sense organs, electrochemical sensory inputs from body tissues and organs, inputs derived from the immune system and inputs that derive from the thinking, analysing and planning centres of the brain, all serve to create specific ANS driving stimuli. Thus, at least in part, the ANS is subservient to the wishes and desires created in our mind. If you want to get up out of the chair and go for a walk—the ANS has to organise the physiological backup and supply networks that support the action demanded.

Figure 1.1, taken from Janig and Habler (1999) and modified slightly, usefully illustrates where the ANS occupancy of the nervous/homeostatic systems sits. The model, which is quite like the Mature Organism Model (Gifford 1998) in that it is 'circular'—having input, processing and output elements—nicely illustrates the integration of all elements of the body including the brain and its higher centres.

The following example may help you/the reader appreciate the role of the ANS and the importance of models like these to clinical reasoning.

In creation of hunger, 'body organs' relay information to the CNS about the levels of glucose in the blood. Information may be via neural or humoral/endocrine systems and messengers. From the neural pathway perspective, it is known that special chemoreceptive sensory nerve fibre endings that respond to blood glucose levels exist in the pancreas and gastrointestinal tract as well as in the blood vessels of the third ventricle of the brain adjacent to the hypothalamus. The 'sampled' information is then relayed to specific regions of the CNS that scrutinise and deal with 'actions' relating to hunger and energy supply. The message is simply—'energy levels low, please restore.' The CNS regions involved in scrutinising and mounting a co-ordinated response are thought to reside in the hypothalamus, in particular, the paraventricular and ventromedial nuclei and the lateral hypothalamic areas (Westmoreland et al 1994). 'Output' from these areas may be directed to the limbic and neocortical areas, creating the sensation of hunger, which in turn drives food gathering behaviour via the musculoskeletal system and thence to the 'external world' as noted in Figure 1.1.

At the same time:

- Autonomic output activates relevant regions of the alimentary tract in order to make ready for food intake and digestion.
- Autonomic activity will also stimulate the pancreas and adrenal glands, both of which are important in the hormonal regulation of glucose and energy metabolism.
- Autonomic activity will co-ordinate the cardiovascular system so that blood supply demands may be met from the musculoskeletal system whose activities are needed to gather food, prepare, eat, and metabolise it.

As the process of food gathering and feeding proceed so the input, scrutinising, and output systems change their activities in response to the changing situations.

25

It is often said that the sympathetic system 'kicks into action during emergencies'. Robert Salposky (1994) adds the (clinically) important caveat 'or what you *think* are emergencies'—that underlines the importance of personal assessment of the situation we find ourselves in. Thus, how the sympathetic system responds is very much influenced by the emotional, cognitive and conscious brain—'our' interpretation of the situation we are in is hugely responsible for its activities. If you believe the pain you have signifies a serious illness or condition you will have a far different 'sympathetic' reaction than if you dismiss the pain and pass it off as trivial. If as a patient you think that what the therapist is doing to you makes sense and feels right you will have quite a different response from someone who might be feeling unsure or even slightly anxious about what is being done to them (see also Chapter 4). It is probable that a clinician's most powerful effect on a patient's sympathetic system activity is produced via the atmosphere of the therapeutic interaction. Importantly, this relates more to what the patient actually feels and interprets, than to what the clinician thinks they should feel or should have interpreted. The effect of a productive 'therapeutic alliance' on the activities of systems like the ANS should never be underestimated (see the Placebo section in Topical Issues in Pain 4.)

Autonomic anatomy—from spinal cord out

As discussed, the sympathetic and parasympathetic systems are efferent—just like the somatic motor system they have an 'effect' on the tissues that they innervate. Simply, impulses radiate from the central nervous system to target tissues in the body. While activity in somatic motor efferent neurones cause striated muscles to contract, those in the autonomic nervous system have a wide range of targets and effects. For example, via the sympathetic innervation of smooth muscles in blood vessel walls sympathetic activity can alter vessel lumen size and hence alter blood flow; it can cause secretory glands to be activated or inactivated; and, via secretion of chemicals from vesicles in its terminals, it can influence the chemical environment, the health and the healing of the tissues innervated (see Chapters 2 and 3). As well as having the capacity to have quite massive effects, it also seems that the autonomic nervous system is capable of acting in a highly specific and localised way.

The sympathetic system

This section is intended to provide the reader with an overview of a poorly understood system. Review of classic anatomical texts and overviews by current leaders in the field of autonomic nervous system anatomy, physiology and function reveals quite marked discrepancies and inconsistencies. The reader would be well advised to read some of the papers and texts cited at the end of this chapter for fuller accounts.

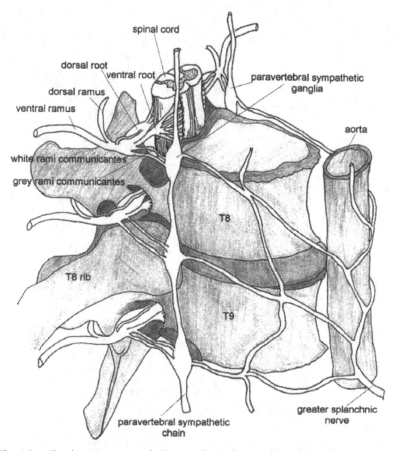

Fig. 1.2   The thoracic paravertebral sympathetic chain and its relationships

Adapted from: Harati Y, Machkhas H 1997 Spinal cord and peripheral nervous system. In: Low PA (ed) Clinical Autonomic Disorders 2nd edn. Lippincott-Raven, Philadelphia

The best known parts of the sympathetic system are the two sympathetic chains or trunks that extend from the base of the skull to the coccyx. These two '**paravertebral**' sympathetic chains lie on either side of the vertebral column (Figs 1.2, 1.3, 1.4 & 1.5) but may come together and fuse in the sacral region to form the ganglion 'impar'. Each chain has about 22 or 23 **paravertebral ganglia** which contain nerve axons and the cell bodies of postganglionic neurones. A ganglion is a swelling of a nerve due to the large numbers of cell bodies it contains. Sympathetic ganglia can be thought of as communication boxes or relay stations where information in the form of impulses may be modulated and passed on, even prevented from passing

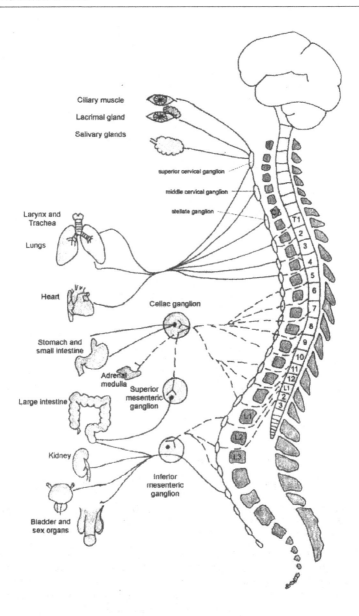

Fig. 1.3 The organisation, layout, relations and basic supply of the peripheral sympathetic system. Dashed lines represent preganglionic fibres, continuous lines represent postganglionic fibres.

Adapted from: Harati Y, Machkhas H 1997 Spinal cord and peripheral nervous system. In: Low PA (ed) Clinical Autonomic Disorders 2nd edn. Lippincott-Raven, Philadelphia

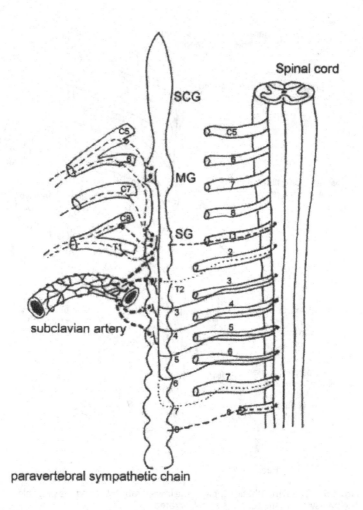

Fig. 1.4 The origin and course of the sympathetic fibres to the arm. The diagram also shows the cervical sympathetic chain, roots and brachial plexus relationships. The preganglionic fibres from T2 and T7 are dotted because their supply to the upper limb is uncertain. The preganglionic fibres from T1 and T8 are dashed to show they are present but not involved in the upper limb sympathetic supply. The cervical roots have no preganglionic fibres and the spinal nerves of the plexus that derive from these roots only have grey rami communicantes. SCG: superior cervical ganglion; MG middle cervical ganglion; SG stellate ganglion.

Adapted from Grieve GP 1994 The autonomic nervous system in vertebral pain syndromes, Fig. 20.4. In: Boyling JD, Palastanga N (eds) Grieve's Modern Manual Therapy 2nd edn. Churchill Livingstone, Edinburgh

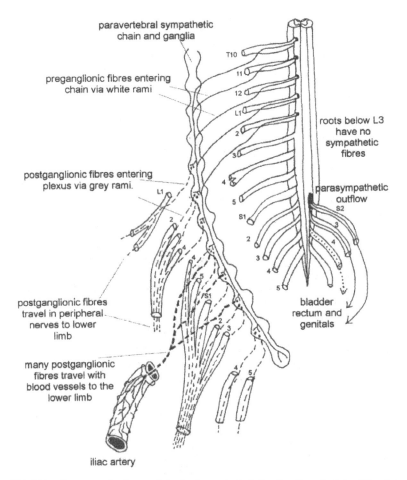

paravertebral sympathetic
chain and ganglia

preganglionic fibres entering
chain via white rami

roots below L3
have no
sympathetic
fibres

postganglionic fibres entering
plexus via grey rami.

parasympathetic
outflow
S2

postganglionic fibres
travel in peripheral
nerves to lower
limb

bladder
rectum and
genitals

many postganglionic
fibres travel with
blood vessels to the
lower limb

iliac artery

Fig. 1.5 The sympathetic supply to the lower limbs following the principle of Fig. 1.4. The parasympathetic supply is also illustrated.

Adapted from Grieve GP 1994 The autonomic nervous system in vertebral pain syndromes, Fig. 20.5. In: Boyling JD, Palastanga N (eds) Grieve's Modern Manual Therapy 2nd edn. Churchill Livingstone, Edinburgh

on, or simply allowed to pass straight through unchecked. Many of the paravertebral ganglia relate to the cord segment from which they derive (Fig. 1.3). However, there are fewer in number than there are segments in the spine as some of the ganglia are fused. In the cervical region there are normally three ganglia—the most rostral being the superior cervical ganglion, below this is the middle cervical, and lowest of all, the stellate ganglia (Figs 1.3, 1.4). The stellate ganglion consists of the fused inferior cervical ganglion with the first thoracic ganglion. There are usually four ganglia in the lumbar part of the chain and four or five in the sacral region.

The spinal cord only connects to the sympathetic chain via the 14 spinal nerves that exit from the intervertebral foramen between T1 and L3 (i.e. via roots T1–L2) (Figs 1.3, 1.4, 1.5). Hence its 'outflow' is said to be 'thoraco-lumbar'. This means that all the peripheral sympathetic nerve pathways to the target tissues and organs of the body have their origins in the spinal cord segments of T1 to L3 (but see Grieve 1994, p 297).

Although it has segmental origins, the SNS, to quite a marked extent, actually defies the traditional description of a segmental system (see below). Thus, sympathetic supply to the head and neck has its origins from *the nerve roots* of T1–T5 (mostly upper 2 or 3); the upper limb from roots T2–T6 (but possibly as far as T7 or T8) (Fig. 1.4); the thorax from roots T3–T6; the abdomen from roots T7–T11 and the lower limbs from roots T10–L2 or L3 (Fig. 1.5).

This supply may be an important consideration when investigating the consequences of thoracic and high lumbar nerve trunk and nerve root injuries or irritations. What can be applauded is the neat fact that these vital control supply lines exit and have their origins from parts of the spinal column that are relatively rarely injured and well protected.

The sympathetic supply involves a two neurone pathway from the spinal cord to the target tissues of the periphery (Fig. 1.6). These neurones are termed *preganglionic* and *postganglionic* respectively.

There is some evidence that the sympathetic ganglia contain inter-neurones, termed 'SIF' (small intensely fluorescent) cells that may serve modulatory functions, i.e. they aid in the integration or processing of incoming and outgoing information (see Grieve 1994, p 299).

The preganglionic neurones of the sympathetic system have their cell bodies in the lateral grey horn (Fig. 1.7), (also known as the intermediate zone, or interomediolateral cell column) of the spinal cord. As already noted, the cell bodies of these neurones are only found in segments T1 to L3 (Westmoreland et al 1994) of the spinal cord. Its segmental origins are worth noting since the sympathetic system innervates just about every tissue of the body via these spinal segments.

Myelinated preganglionic fibres pass away from the spinal cord via the ventral root and into the spinal nerve for a short distance, then via the *white* rami communicantes they join the sympathetic trunk.

Having reached the sympathetic trunk, the preganglionic sympathetic fibres may do several things (see Fig. 1.7). Some synapse with postganglionic cells in the *paravertebral* ganglion that lies at the same level from which they exit the vertebral column (nos 1, 3 & 4 in Fig. 1.7). Others pass through their segmental ganglion and run up or down to more distant *paravertebral* ganglia where they terminate and synapse with postganglionic fibres (no. 5 in Fig. 1.7). Note how this defies the idea of 'segmentalism'. It is commonly stated that there is a pre to postganglionic neurone divergence ratio of anything from 1:1 to 1:196 (see Grieve 1994, Williams et al 1995). In other words one preganglionic fibre may terminate with only one postganglionic fibre, or may have a massive terminal aborisation connecting to a great many. The

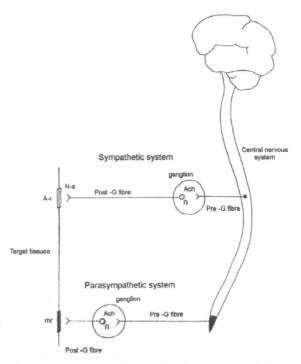

Fig. 1.6 The basic arrangement of the peripheral components of the sympathetic and parasympathetic systems. Note the long to short relationship of the pre to post ganglionic sympathetic fibres and the opposite for the parasympathetic fibres. Cranial outflow of the parasympathetic system not illustrated here. Classic neurotransmitters and receptor types for each system are illustrated: **A-r** adrenoreceptor; **mr** muscarinic receptor; **n** nicotinic receptor; **N-a** noradrenaline/norepinephrine; **Ach** acetylcholine.

reality is that there is anatomical *convergence* (many preganglionic fibres going to one postganglionic fibre), as well as anatomical *divergence* (the opposite). Importantly, anatomical convergence / divergence does not mean that all the connections are necessarily always functional. Just as elsewhere in the nervous system, there is a huge potential for a spread of effect or a focus of effect that is dependent on continuously fluctuating inhibitory and excitatory modulatory controls. This attribute allows for both expansion and exquisite refinement of autonomic outputs and argues against the blind acceptance of the generalised fight and flight-related function of this system. The possible modulatory role of ganglionic inter-neurones as well as branches from returning visceral sensory afferents (see below) may be important here.

What we do know is that the SNS tends to be a *functionally* 'divergent' system—where small numbers of preganglionic fibres have the potential to influence larger numbers of postganglionic fibres—hence the potential for a single 'action' message producing far reaching effects on target organs and

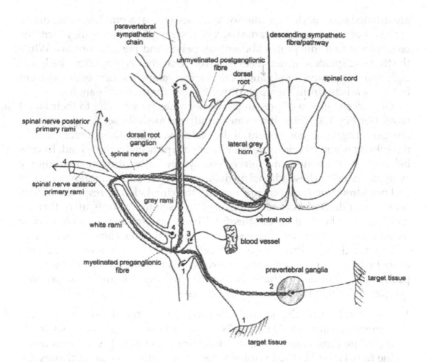

Fig. 1.7 Diagrammatic representation of the various 'pathways' the sympathetic system can take from the thoracic cord to the periphery. Refer to text for details of nos 1–5.

Adapted from: Harati Y, Machkhas H 1997 Spinal cord and peripheral nervous system. In: Low PA (ed) Clinical Autonomic Disorders 2nd edn. Lippincott-Raven, Philadelphia

tissues. The fact that there may be provision for control of this divergence helps explain a degree of specificity, too.

In a similar way to that described in the CNS, the potential for excessive reactivity and spread of effect due to maladaptively altered modulatory controls, or even loss of control, having far reaching effects on sympathetic activity seems a reasonable possibility. Clinically this may provide a possible explanation for reports of localised patches of skin colour change, or localised sweating or swelling disturbances that spread to larger areas over time.

Many preganglionic fibres pass right through the sympathetic chain and paravertebral ganglia without synapsing on postganglionic fibre cells at all (no. 2 in Fig. 1.7). These continue out of the sympathetic chains in the *splanchnic* nerves to reach remote ganglia situated nearer their target organs. These more distant ganglia are often called '**prevertebral' ganglia** (Figs 1.3, 1.7). Well known prevertebral ganglia supplied via the *thoracic* splanchnic nerves are the *celiac, superior* and *inferior mesenteric* ganglia. These ganglia are situated in the abdomen anterior to the abdominal aorta close to the origin of the celiac and mesenteric arteries. Via postganglionic fibres they form the *celiac plexus* that innervates abdominal, pelvic and perineal organs. While the thoracic splanchnic nerves derive from branches arising from the lower eight thoracic *paravertebral* ganglia, the *lumbar* splanchnic nerves derive from branches arising from the upper three lumbar *paravertebral* ganglia.

One special group of preganglionic neurones pass *directly* to their target tissue (see Fig. 1.3). These innervate the adrenal medulla, seemingly omitting the 'postganglionic' component of the pathway. In fact, the adrenal medulla resembles nervous tissue more than it does a typical endocrine gland. Its cells behave like neurones and derive embryologically from postganglionic sympathetic cells. These adrenal medulla cells secrete adrenaline (epinephrine) and noradrenaline (norepinephrine) into the circulation in response to SNS activity that derives from situations that are exciting or stressful, or that are anticipated to be exciting or stressful. This is an excellent example of how mind influences body and can easily be translated to the clinical encounter!

Postganglionic fibres have their cell bodies in the autonomic ganglia described above. Their *unmyelinated* axons radiate to the target tissues. Those postganglionic fibres that have their origins in the ganglia of the *paravertebral* sympathetic chain follow three main courses:

1. Pass back into the spinal somatic nerve trunk via grey rami communicantes (no. 4 in Fig. 1.7). Some apparently may pass back in via the white rami communicantes, too (Janig & Habler 1999). From there, the fibres travel in the peripheral nerves to supply the target tissues, for example, the blood vessels (vasomotor), and sweat glands (sudomotor) in the territories of the nerves they accompany. Thus, postganglionic axons from the cervical ganglia innervate upper extremity tissues by entering the cervical spinal nerves of the brachial plexus deriving from C4–C8, and following the peripheral nerve trunks (see Fig. 1.4). Grey rami communicantes in the neck may pierce and travel through the longus capitis or the scalenus anterior muscles—a fact that may be an important consideration in whiplash injury (see Thacker 1998). Clearly, if these grey rami are injured it may mean the loss of sympathetic supply and control to blood vessels and tissues of the arm.

2. Pass to blood vessels in the neighbourhood of the sympathetic trunk (no. 3 in Figs 1.7 and 1.2, 1.4, & 1.5) and supply these or travel along with them to reach more distal targets. For example, axons from the superior cervical ganglion innervate the pupil of the eye and provide sweat gland innervation of the face by following the course of branches of the internal and external carotid arteries to get there.

3. Pass to visceral organs. For example, postganglionic fibres whose origins are in the lower cervical and upper thoracic ganglia innervate the heart via the cardiac plexus to produce cardiac stimulation, or reach the tracheobrachial tree via the pulmonary plexus to control bronchodilation (we need more efficient lungs when we are about to perform physically, e.g. as in competition or combat).

Postganglionic fibres may pass to higher or lower levels within the sympathetic trunk before leaving via the above routes. For example, although we traditionally describe the efferent supply to the arm as arising from C4–C8 it may be from as low as T7 or T8 if we trace the sympathetic supply back to the roots and spinal cord.

Clinical implications

Some clinically related points:

1. It is important to emphasise that all peripheral nerves contain sympathetic post ganglionic fibres and that they enter the nerves via grey rami communicantes.

This means that those somatic nerves that derive from nerve roots above T1 (including many cranial nerves) and from roots of L3 and below, still receive their supply via grey rami communicantes but will have no white rami communicantes (Figs 1.4 & 1.5). Think about it and you realise that all the cervical nerve *roots* and those roots below L3 will have *no* sympathetic neurones. The sympathetic nerve fibres join the spinal nerves *outside* the intervertebral foramen. This may well be an important clinical/diagnostic consideration. For example, it may explain the common clinical finding that classic acute and sub-acute nerve root disorders in these regions show no signs of classic 'sympathetic abnormality' when compared to patients with symptoms attributable to nerve injury beyond the root level, or from levels where roots contain sympathetic fibres. It has been suggested that the tortuous routes taken by sympathetic fibres may in itself present a greater potential for trauma and irritation (Pick 1970).

2. As stated earlier, the cervical ganglia contain preganglionic fibres that may have their origins from nerve roots as low as T8.

This means that injuries or irritations of nerve roots in the upper and middle thoracic regions can have effects in the arms and head as well as in the viscera and somatic tissues more locally. Clinical investigations of upper extremity oedema, skin health, changes in circulation, changes in temperature or sweating must consider possible root origins in the thoracic spine.

3. The major sympathetic vasoconstrictor supply to the upper limb arteries derives from roots T2 and T3.

The vasoconstrictor supply reaches the upper limb arteries via branches from the brachial plexus. This beautifully illustrates the complex anatomical routing of the sympathetic supply—from spinal cord, to ventral root of T2 and T3, into the ventral ramus, out via the white rami communicantes into the sympathetic chain—then synapsing with postganglionic fibres that course into the brachial plexus via grey rami communicantes before continuing on in the peripheral nerves to their vascular destinations. Changes in skin temperature and circulatory perfusion of the arm associated with musculoskeletal disorders like the chronic regional pain syndromes (CRPS I and II) may well relate to modest nerve injuries or irritations whose origins are in the upper thoracic regions.

Many postganglionic fibres that derive from the stellate ganglion supply the vasoconstrictor and sudomotor supply to the head; secretory fibres to the salivary glands; the pupil dilator muscles and muscles in the upper and lower eyelids.

Recall 'Horners syndrome' that results from destruction of this ganglion. Horner's syndrome is characterised by constriction of the pupil, drooping of the upper eyelid (ptosis), enophthalmos (recession of the eyeball within the orbit) and absence of sweating on the face and neck. It is advisable for clinicians to seek out information relating to the face and eyes following significant neck traumas like whiplash.

Patients who have had simple tissue injuries, nerve injuries, spinal injuries or sprains/strains and some patients with symptoms classified as nerve root irritations quite often report symptoms and signs that are puzzling and not easy to explain. Knowledge of the complex innervation and workings of the sympathetic supply to the head, arms and legs can greatly help us, and often the patient too, to understand the possible origins of odd and understandably worrying symptoms. Common examples include: those related to temperature changes, changes in circulation, skin coloration, abnormal localised sweating, apparent and actual feelings of swelling, skin changes, visual disturbances, and dry mouth. Skilled clinicians may well ask about these types of symptoms in appropriate cases—and in so doing help to reassure the patient that what they describe is quite logical and reasonable when known anatomical features are taken into consideration.

Clinicians should also be on guard against an assumption of neural pathology when these types of symptoms are reported. For example it is well known that some patients with chronic pain syndromes demonstrate increased levels of somatic awareness. Patients are often anxious about their condition and their pain, more especially if they have been given an inadequate examination and explanation by those who the patient feels should know. The result can be that the patients' attention becomes increasingly focused on sensations from their body, many which are either normal but are interpreted as abnormal or else relate to the physical manifestations of their distress. Clinicians are urged to be aware that symptoms of distress/anxiety often present in musculoskeletal tissues—for example many people when they are stressed get pain across the base of the neck and shoulders or in the low back.

In thoracic spinal injuries and presentations thought to have origins in the thoracic spine it is worth considering the SNS supply to the viscera and legs, and hence the potential for dysfunction in the relevant organs and tissues. Here again, enquiries about digestive, excretory and sexual function may be appropriate.

The sympathetic supply to the lower limb has its origins from T10, T11, T12 and L1–L2 occasionally L3 segments of the spinal cord. These spinal levels may be justifiably considered as possible sources in patients reporting 'sympathetic' effects in the lower limbs.

In all cases where the label 'sympathetic' symptoms is a possibility, great caution is advised in jumping to conclusions about pathology, pathological sources, symptom mechanisms and interventions. There is insufficient supportive evidence to pinpoint blame on the SNS unequivocally (see Chapters 2–5).

The effects of sympathetic and parasympathetic activity on target organs are summarised in Table 1.1.

The parasympathetic system

The traditional concept of the parasympathetic system is that it has an opposite and antagonistic effect to sympathetic activity on the organs and tissues innervated. However, Janig and Habler (1999) indicate that this state of affairs is the exception rather than the rule. In their overview of both systems (see Table 1.1) they state that:

- Most target *tissues* react only to one of the systems—the pacemaker cells of the heart are the exception.
- A few *organs* react to both—e.g., the iris, heart and urinary bladder.
- Most effects of both systems are excitatory, inhibition being rare.

Where there is reciprocal effect of the two systems on the target cells, it can usually be shown either that the systems work synergistically or that they exert their influence under different functional conditions. Two examples serve to illustrate this:

a) the opposite actions of sympathetic and parasympathetic systems on the size of the pupil is a consequence of the separate target cells supplied by each system – i.e. they go to different muscles;
b) fast changes of heart rate during changes of body position and emotional stress are generated via changes in activity in the parasympathetic neurons to the pacemaker cells; the sustained increase of heart rate during exercise is mainly generated by activation of sympathetic neurons supplying the heart.

Because the parasympathetic system's supply to its target tissues and organs is via four cranial nerves and nerves that have their origins in the second, third and fourth sacral nerves, the parasympathetic system is said to have a 'craniosacral outflow' (Figs 1.8, 1.5). Like the sympathetic system, the parasympathetic pathway consists of two neurones—a pre and postganglionic, with synapsing occurring between the two in parasympathetic ganglia. But unlike the sympathetic system, which mostly has short preganglionic and long postganglionic fibres, the parasympathetic system has very long preganglionic fibres. The postganglionic fibres tend to be short and derive from many very small ganglia that lie very close, or actually in, the target tissues. The ratio of pre to postganglionic fibres is between 1:15 and 1:20. Figure 1.8 summarises the supply.

Table 1.1 Effects of activation of sympathetic and parasympathetic neurones on autonomic target organs. (Adapted from Janig & Habler 1999)

Organ and organ system	Activation of parasympathetic nerves	Activation of sympathetic nerves
Heart muscle	Decrease of heart rate	Increase of heart rate
	Decrease of contractility	Increase of contractility
	(only atria)	(atria, ventricles)
Blood vessels		
Arteries		
In skin of trunk and limbs	0	Vasoconstriction
In skin and mucosa of face	Vasodilation	Vasoconstriction
In visceral domain	0	Vasoconstriction
In skeletal muscle	0	Vasoconstriction
		Vasodilation (cholinergic)
In heart (coronary arteries)		Vasoconstriction
In erectile tissue	Vasodilation	Vasoconstriction
In cranium	Vasodilation (?)	Vasoconstriction
Veins	0	Vasoconstriction
Gastrointestinal tract		
Longitudinal and circular muscle	Increase of motility	Decrease in motility
Sphincters	Relaxation	Contraction
Capsule of spleen	0	Contraction
Urinary bladder		
Detrusor vesicae	Contraction	Relaxation (small)
Trigone (internal sphincter)	0	Contraction
Reproductive organs		
Seminal vesicle, prostate	0	Contraction
Vas deferens	0	Contraction
Uterus	0	Contraction
		Relaxation — depends on species and hormonal state.
Eye		
Dilator muscle of pupil	0	Contraction (mydriasis)
Sphincter muscle of pupil	Contraction (miosis)	0
Ciliary muscle	Contraction (accomodation)	
Tarsal muscle	0	Contraction (lifting of lid)
Orbital muscle	0	Contraction (protrusion of eye)
Tracheo-bronchial muscles	Contraction	Relaxation (probably mainly by adrenaline)
Piloerector muscles	0	Contraction
Exocrine glands		
Salivary glands	Copious secretion	Weak mucous secretion
Lachrymal glands	Secretion	0
Nasopharyngeal glands	Secretion	
Bronchial glands	Secretion	?
Sweat glands	0	Secretion (cholinergic)
Digestive glands (stomach, pancreas)	Secretion	Decrease of secretion or 0
Mucosa (small, large intestine)	Secretion	Decrease of secretion or reabsorption
Pineal gland	0	Increase in synthesis of melatonin
Brown and adipose tissue	0	Heat production
Metabolism		
Liver	0	Glycogenolysis, glucongeogenesis
Fat cells	0	Lipolysis (free fatty acids in blood increased)
β-cells in islets of pancreas	Secretion	Decrease in secretion of pancreas
Adrenal medulla	0	Secretion of adrenaline and noradrenaline
Lymphoid tissue	0	Depression of activity (e.g. of natural killer cells)

Some key nerves that contain parasympathetic innervation:

Oculomotor supply (cranial nerve III). The preganglionic fibres travel in the oculomotor nerve to the *ciliary ganglia*. Short postganglionic fibres supply the muscles of the eye and control lens focusing via the ciliary muscles.

Facial parasympathetic supply (cranial nerve VII). The facial nerve sends preganglionic fibres to two major ganglia—the *pterygopalatine* and the *submandibular*. The pterygopalatine postganglionic fibres supply glands in the lining of the mouth and nose and the tear glands. They also supply vasodilatory and secretory input to arteries, veins and glands of the face, nose, mouth, tongue, eyes and cerebrum. The postganglionic innervation deriving from the submandibular ganglia gives rise to a stimulatory supply to the submandibular and sublingual glands (salivary).

Glossopharyngeal parasympathetic supply (cranial nerve IX). Preganglionic fibres run to the *otic* ganglia that via its postganglionic fibres supplies the parotid gland. Some postganglionic neurons may also supply blood vessels of the jaw, the cerebral circulation and sweat glands around the lips.

Vagus parasympathetic supply (cranial nerve X). This dramatic nerve leaves the skull via the jugular foramen with the same dural sleeve as the glossopharyngeal and accessory nerves and descends into the abdomen. Its efferent parasympathetic supply is summarised in Figure 1.8.

Sacral parasympathetic outflow. Preganglionic fibres pass from the spinal cord segments S2–S4 to the ventral rami of the nerve roots. The fibres then pass within the roots down the spinal canal and out of their respective ventral foramen on the sacrum where they join to form the various branches and nerves of the sacral plexus. Parasympathetic supply leaves the sacral plexus as the pelvic splanchnic nerves. These nerves join the hypogastric plexus that derives from the pelvic part of the sympathetic chain. The sacral parasympathetic fibres supply the distal colon, rectum, bladder, prostate, kidney, sex organs and external genitalia. (Fig. 1.8)

Those readers who wish to know more about urogenital nerve supply and urogenital pain syndromes in men and women are advised to consult Wesselmann's work (Wesselmann 1999, Wesselmann 2000).

Neurotransmitters and receptors of the ANS

The nervous system specialises in sending information—fast. Fast transmission of information involves impulses as a result of action potentials along the length of the axon. Where axons end they form synapses with other neurones or communicate with their target tissues via 'neuroeffector' junctions. The fast electrical message that arrives at the end of the axon produces its effect by stimulating the release of chemical messenger agents called neurotransmitters (see Fig. 1.6).

In the autonomic nervous system the peripheral pathway involves two neurones and therefore a single synapse between the dendrites of the

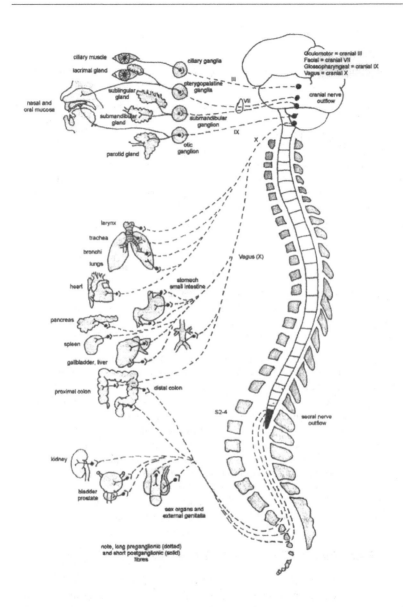

Fig. 1.8 The organisation, layout, relations and basic supply of the peripheral parasympathetic system. Dashed lines represent preganglionic fibres, continuous lines represent postganglionic fibres.

Adapted from: Harati Y, Machkhas H 1997 Spinal cord and peripheral nervous system. In: Low PA (ed) Clinical Autonomic Disorders 2nd edn. Lippincott-Raven, Philadelphia preganglionic neurones and the ganglionic cell body of the postganglionic neurones (see Fig. 1.6). Preganglionic neurones of all sympathetic and parasympathetic neurones are said to be *cholinergic* because the neurotransmitter they liberate following the arrival of an action potential is acetylcholine. Acetylcholine then diffuses across the synaptic cleft and binds to receptor molecules on the cell membrane of the postganglionic cell body. This receptor binding process causes adjacent ion channels to open and a flow of ions to occur across the cell membrane. The resultant flow of ions across the cell membrane gives rise to a change in membrane voltage which in turn leads to the formation of a post synaptic action potential that then forms the impulse radiating to the nerve ends of the postganglionic fibre in the target tissues. The predominant acetylcholine receptor molecules in the postganglionic cell membrane are called *nicotinic* receptors, so named because the excitatory effect can be imitated by locally applied nicotine.

The end terminals of the postganglionic nerve are often termed neuroeffector junctions. Here, the junctions of sympathetic and parasympathetic systems differ in the chemical transmitters they secrete.

All postganglionic neurones contain large numbers of varicosities ('bags' containing the neurotransmitters) strung along the axon branches where they are in contact with the target organ tissue. The chief sympathetic postganglionic neurone transmitter substance is norepinephrine (noradrenaline)—hence the sympathetic system in general is described as *adrenergic*. The parasympathetic neurone, on the other hand secretes acetylcholine—hence the term *cholinergic*.

In the case of the sympathetic system, noradrenaline is released in to the tissues and causes its effects there via noradrenaline receptors expressed on the tissues it supplies. These receptors are usually referred to as 'adrenoreceptors' and there are many 'subtypes' now known.

Adrenoreceptors may be found:

- On the cells of the tissues innervated.
- On any immune cells that may be present.
- On smooth muscle cells in local vasculature.
- On any sensory cells in the area, for example nociceptors.
- On the sympathetic terminals themselves—hence noradrenaline may be released by the sympathetic terminal and then act on it to produce further activity.

This 'self stimulation' is termed an autocrine effect. For example, there is now a good body of research demonstrating that released noradrenaline acts on adjacent adrenoreceptors on the postganglionic terminals to cause the production and release of prostaglandins that may cause nociceptor sensitisation or even pain (see Levine & Reichling 1999; see also Chapters 2–4).

An important principle for the clinician is to appreciate that any transmitter chemical like noradrenaline can only have an effect on a target tissue if active and relevant receptors for the chemical are present. Appreciate also, that chemical agents that activate the receptors are called 'agonists' and that 'antagonists' block the receptors and hence prevent their activity. Phentolamine, discussed in Chapter 4, is an example of an adrenoreceptor antagonist commonly used in the diagnosis and management of sympathetically maintained pain.

Readers interested in a more detailed account of the neurochemical organisation of the autonomic nervous system are advised to consult Milner et al (1999).

The enteric nervous system—the brain of the gut

The enteric nervous system is peculiar to the gastrointestinal tract and consists of a network of nerve cells and fibres embedded in its walls. It is considered to be a semiautonomous system with specific 'programmes' for motor responses, such as peristaltic reflexes and regional rate of contraction via its pacemaker systems (Camilleri 1997).

It consists of two major plexuses, the *myenteric (Auerbach's)* and the *submucous (Meissner's)* plexuses. There are also plexuses of nerve-fibre bundles in the muscle layers, mucosa, subserosa and around arteries. It is surprising to consider that there may be as many nerve cell bodies in the gut as there are in the spinal cord, about 100 million!! Further details can be found in Camilleri (1997).

According to Camilleri (1997), the current concept is that the enteric nerve complex has integrative sensory, interneurone and motor systems that can function independently of sympathetic and parasympathetic input from the CNS. It is believed that there are 'hard-wired' modules that detect the chemical and physical condition and contents of the gut, process the information in well established inter-neurone circuits and then mount appropriate motor responses involving control of secretory tissues and organs as well as muscular activity. Inputs from the CNS via the parasympathetic and sympathetic systems are thought to modulate the response patterns, and may even be able to 'select' particular responses to suit conditions elsewhere. CNS control is via the 'excitatory' parasympathetic vagal pathway on the one hand, and the sympathetic pathways that function to inactivate and inhibit gut muscle and digestive activities on the other.

The clinical message is that when under stress, threat or when life gets exciting, gut 'activity' and digestion is inhibited or even shut down—since it wastes vital energy that would otherwise be useful for survival. During stress our digestive secretions dry up (water conservation) and peristalsis halts. Diarrhoea associated with acute stress indicates however that one end of the system is active! From an evolutionary perspective (see Sapolsky 1994) this short lived event is a very adaptive strategy: first, clearing out the lower bowel (and bladder too) lightens the load to enable escape/more efficient action in the face of physical threat and second it makes you far less palatable to any predator due to the noxious smell and rather unsightly mess! The detrimental effects of ongoing stress are likely to include negative effects on bowel function—hence conditions like irritable bowel syndrome (reviewed in Chaitow 2000) that often occur concurrently in patients with chronic pain disability.

In times of low stress levels the gut is left unhindered to function efficiently. Patients with ongoing pain states, or who have pain states that are a source of high concern, are often highly distressed. The impact of this kind of ongoing and unresolved stress response on gut function and gut health is likely to be negative.

The visceral sensory system—the 'autonomic or visceral afferents'

The viscera contains terminals of sensory neurones and very definitely has a sensory innervation (see e.g. Janig & Habler 1995). Visceral afferents may be mechanosensitive—being activated by various types of mechanical distortion (think bladder, gut, lungs and blood pressure) or chemically, for example picking up the osmolarity of the blood, or the concentrations of glucose. Some afferents may only be excited when the tissues are inflamed and therefore signal noxious events. Interestingly, vagal afferents innervating the liver may signal information in relation to toxins/infections picked up from the blood and as a result mediate general and protective sickness behaviours which includes a generalised increase in physical sensitivity (i.e. hyperalgesia) (Watkins et al 1995, Pennisi 1997, Sternberg & Gold 1997, Watkins 1997). It is certainly common to feel physically stiff and generally uncomfortable when you are suffering with an infection or are feeling unwell. Minor knocks and bumps can often be sickeningly painful. It seems a reasonable evolutionary tactic for the brain to put the somatic sensory systems on higher alert when we are in a more vulnerable state. Consider also that many patients in pain are well below 'par' and may already be nudged towards a hyperalgesic state. Add to this the toxic effects of medications and further shifts may occur.

Afferent fibres from the viscera travel to the central nervous system in the nerves and nerve plexuses described above for the sympathetic and parasympathetic systems. Thus, visceral afferents are found in the vagus and glossopharyngeal nerves and possibly other cranial nerves; also they are found in the second, third and fourth sacral nerves and in the thoracic and upper lumbar spinal nerves. Visceral sensory fibres can be divided into three types:

1. **Visceral afferents** that project to the **spinal cord** (Fig. 1.9). Like their somatic counterparts these visceral sensory fibres have their cell bodies in the dorsal root ganglia and their central terminals in the outer lamina of the cord dorsal horn. These 'spinal' afferents travel from the viscera mainly in the splanchnic nerves and amount to only 1.5–2.0% of all spinal afferents that have their cell bodies in the dorsal root ganglia (Janig &

Habler 1995). Clearly, the viscera has a relatively poor sensory supply when compared to the skin, where the supply is vast, or the deep somatic domain, where it is more modest than the skin, but still significant compared to the gut. As discussed below visceral primary afferents may send collateral branches to sympathetic postganglionic efferents in the prevertebral ganglia.

2. **Visceral afferents** that travel to the CNS via **cranial nerves** and terminate in appropriate brain nuclei. For example, central endings of afferents travelling in the vagus nerve mainly terminate in the nucleus of the solitary tract (NST) that lies in the brain stem. Ritter et al (1992) state that 80–85% of nerve fibres in the vagus nerve are afferent fibres.

    Just like somatic sensory fibres, there are several functional subtypes of spinal and cranial visceral afferents. These are discussed in relation to visceral pain in the section following.

3. **'Enteric' visceral afferents** (Fig. 1.9). These afferents lie in the walls of the gut and communicate with enteric interneurones and motor neurones as well as sending branches to prevertebral ganglia where they synapse with postganglionic fibres of the autonomic system.

Visceral primary afferents continually sample the state of affairs in their target organs. Hence information about such things as the contents of the gut, bladder, colon, and the chemistry of the blood may be relayed centrally for processing and the generation of appropriate responses. Higher centres and 'consciousness' may become involved; we well know that situations in the viscera often promote physical action, such as when our bladder or bowel is full, when we are dehydrated, when we are hungry or satiated, and when sexually aroused. However, for many of the mundane operations that go on in the gut there is little need for conscious or subconscious analysis. Much activity and control goes on far nearer the tissues themselves.

Several 'levels' of integrative control have been identified:

1. At the *lowest* integrative control level sits the enteric nervous system of the gut. Here, the neural organisation illustrates its isolated 'sample — scrutinise — response' capabilities and hence, its special autonomy.

2. A *second* integrative level consists of a local control loop involving postganglionic autonomic fibres. Here, collateral branches of centrally projecting primary afferents as well as projections from visceral afferents of the enteric system (Fig. 1.9) synapse with postganglionic sympathetic fibres in the prevertebral ganglia. Hence, the formation of an 'extraspinal' reflex feedback loop. Regulation at this level is said to be via 'extracentral reflexes' since they can operate without involving the CNS, though they may well be influenced by modulating central inputs. These reflexes are thought to be important in control and regulation of gut motility (enhancement of peristalsis, storage function), regulation of fluid (excretion), as well as in protection. 'Protection' or protective reflexes that

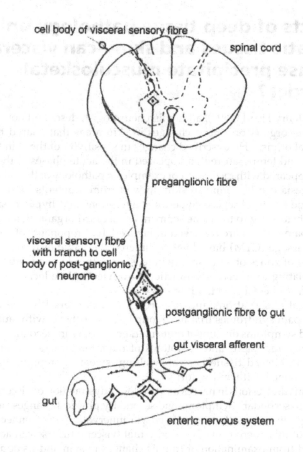

Fig. 1.9 The enteric nervous system and the afferent and efferent pathways between the gut and the spinal cord. Note how the postganglionic fibre activity can be modulated by visceral afferents going to the spinal cord as well as by gut visceral afferents that send branches to the postganglionic cell body.

Adapted from: Janig J, Habler, HJ 1995 Visceral-autonomic integration. In: Gebhart GF (ed) Visceral Pain. Progress in Pain Research and Management Vol. 5. IASP Press, Seattle

inhibit intestinal reflex activity might occur in relation to such things as inflammation of organs, peritonitis, overdistension or obstruction. Similar reflex pathways may also operate in the gall bladder and pancreas (Janig & Habler 1995).

3. Visceral primary afferents are important for *higher level* integration involving reflex segmental spinal and cranial pathways as well as higher CNS processing and outputs.

Effects of deep tissue pathology on somatic tissues and skin—can visceral disease precipitate musculosketal disorder?

In 1893 Henry Head (1893), an English neurologist, described how diseases of internal organs produced changes in skin areas that shared the same segmental origins. He described changes in sensitivity of the skin to touch, pressure and temperature that appeared in the acute phases of the disease and disappeared with recovery. For example, in pathology of the gall bladder, hyperalgesia can be found in skin derived from segments T6–T10. Later, Mackenzie (1909) observed hypertonic alterations and hypersensitivity in muscles belonging to the same segment as diseased organs. Some common sites of pain referral are reviewed in Figure 1.10. Proponents of connective tissue massage (CTM) have long considered the value of recognition and treatment of zones of abnormality in tension in the skin and subcutaneous layers relating to visceral dysfunction (reviewed in Luedecke 1969, Ebner 1975, Gifford J & Gifford L S 1988).

Clinical observations and research into disorders like the complex regional pain syndromes that have long been associated with 'autonomic' signs and symptoms document quite marked changes in 'secondary' tissues. Hence 'referred' signs and symptoms of pain, tenderness (hyperalgesia/ allodynia), altered tissue health, swelling, sweating, temperature, joint function, bone health and so forth.

It seems that lesions in nerves or pathology/dysfunction of visceral organs can lead to secondary symptoms and secondary physical changes, and hence pathology, in tissues that are related via innervation and connectivity. In support of this, there is even evidence that 'visceral disease can actually be predicted from examination of trophic changes in skin and its appendages, subcutis, joint capsules, and fascia...with a probability of about 70%' (Janig & Habler 1995.)

Multiple theories abound (see Janig & Habler 1995), most focusing round the concept that these secondary changes stem from the negative impact of ongoing activity in viscero-sympathetic reflex arcs. Research summarised by Janig and Habler (1995) demonstrates that increased visceral afferent activity from a cat's bladder will cause a segmentally related *increase* in activity of sympathetic efferents involved in skin sweating and muscle circulation and a *decrease* in activity in sympathetic efferents responsible for skin circulation. Thus, noxious input due to excessive distension of the bladder, or experimental inflammation of it, causes increased activity in all visceral afferent fibre types. This includes nociceptors. This activity bears a direct relation to activity in the segmentally related sympathetic efferent fibres that control sweating and circulation. The findings show that noxious input produces a significant decrease in circulation to muscles, an increase in sweating and an increase in circulation to the skin. The research also demonstrates significant ongoing activity for several hours after the provocation abates. It is not difficult to envisage that ongoing activity of days or weeks could lead to prolonged changes in circulation leading to trophic and other changes in the tissues affected. For example, prolonged increases in circulation to skin could result in oedema and prolonged circulatory deprivation to muscle could cause muscle fibre degeneration, dysfunction and impairment.

The disciples of a holistic approach to pain and health have been around for a long time; the evidence that they are right is only now emerging. One system's health or ill-health appears to have the potential to significantly impact traditionally unrelated tissues.

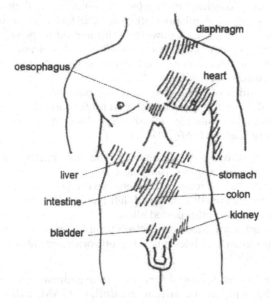

Fig. 1.10 Shaded areas show zones of pain referral felt when organs indicated are diseased/inflamed.

Adapted from: Westmorland et al 1994 Medical Neurosciences 3rd edn. Little Brown, Boston

The autonomic innervation of the immune system, stress and mind-body links

One area of recent interest to mind body pathways and the science of psychoneuroimmunology is the finding that tissues where immune cells develop have a rich autonomic innervation (Watkins 1997). This innervation has been given little attention by pain researchers, yet it may be of considerable relevance.

Thus, sympathetic and parasympathetic fibres are found in bone marrow, the thymus gland and lymphoid tissue and organs generally. It seems that the activity of both branches of the autonomic nervous system have the capacity to modulate the maturity and activation of the immune cells, especially in those areas like the airways and gut that are exposed to antigens and allergens. Watkins (1997) states: 'Although the exact role of autonomic innervation in regulating immunity has not been clearly defined, there is sufficient evidence to suggest that autonomic nerves are capable of regulating almost all the cells involved in inflammation.'

There is some evidence to suggest that age-related dysfunction of the ANS, including that to the lymphoid tissue, may be responsible for the age-related decay in immunological function (see references in Watkins 1997 p. 17). One message is that we should look after our ANS for as long as we can!

Since the activity of the ANS is powerfully influenced by perception of our circumstances, by emotions and by our mood state, this physical linking to the immune system holds interest to those who embrace the need for multidimensional models of health and disease.

The scientific scrutiny of mind-body links and pathways is gathering a great deal of useful and interesting information for the multidimensionally comfortable clinician. For example, in discussing the evidence for cortical control of immunity Watkins (1997 p.17) reports:

- That the effects of stress, perception and personality on immunity have all been extensively investigated (see below.)
- That there appears to be a relationship between cerebral dominance and allergy and auto-immune disease—with left handers having a 11.5-fold increase in incidence of self-reported allergy.
- Lesions of the cortex produced by electrolytic ablation have shown that immunity is suppressed with lesions to the left cortex and enhanced with ablations to the right!

Stress is known to activate central nervous system pathways that mediate the activity of the sympathetic adreno–medullary (SAM) axis—hence increasing levels of circulating adrenaline, as well as the hypothalamic–pituitary–adreno-cortex (HPA) axis that results in increased levels of the circulating steroid cortisol. It has long been postulated that ongoing stress, and hence the effects mediated by these hormones or via the direct pathways detailed above, may have detrimental effects and even produce or promote somatic disease processes as well as changes in mood (e.g. Selye & Tuchweber 1976, Selye 1978, Sapolsky 1994, Martin 1997, Watkins 1997). While fluctuations in stress are a normal part of everyday life and something that evolution has catered for, ongoing stress with no let up is not.

Some points

Stressful situations activate the SAM axis resulting in the fight or flight response and associated feelings of anger and anxiety.

In contrast, activation of the HPA axis promotes submission, and the emotions of defeat and despair. Typically, chronically stressful situations promote a vacillation between anger and despair as individuals fight to gain control over their situation or give up, believing they have no control. 'These cycles of anger and despair promote the production of a destructive range of catabolic hormones, injurious to a number of bodily systems, not just the immune system' (see Watkins 1997, p11).

Animal studies have demonstrated immunosuppresive effects of a wide range of stressors, for example, isolation, separation, overcrowding, introduction of an aggressive intruder, restraint, cold, noise and inescapable foot shock (see Watkins 1997). It seems relatively easy to see the possible links to patients who suffer with ongoing pain syndromes.

Chronic stress has been shown to impair wound healing in humans. Death of a spouse suppresses the immune system for 2–6 weeks. Traumatic marital separation has been shown to be even more immunosuppresive than bereavement. However, Watkins (1997), states that 'current opinion now believes that minor chronic stress, termed "microstress," is more immunosuppresive than single life events such as bereavement.'

In contrast, animal studies have shown increased survival of animals exposed to influenza virus who also underwent restraint stress. The way a stressor is perceived, or the 'will to survive' may have a huge impact on whether there is a positive or negative impact on the immune system or other potentially destructive processes that stress can precipitate. Clinically, the key may be to improve patients' ability to cope, and increase their feelings of control and of self-esteem. If patients are unable to learn the skills that are needed to pick themselves up, and if they continue to see their situation as hopeless, then successful outcomes are unlikely. It seems that the 'will to survive' or at least a positive belief in one's ability to cope, get control, or overcome a situation may have a significant multidimensional health promoting impact.

With response to stress, there is a great inter-individual variability and a marked spectrum to consider. What scares you or makes you feel cautious may not necessarily have the same effect on the next person. But also, what scares you now may not scare you in the future, and what doesn't bother you now, may well do so in years to come. Past experiences, our inborn temperament and our learned and instinctive coping strategies may all have a part to play in how we cope right now.

There is some evidence that psychosocial disruption in utero, postnatally, and during childhood can have long-term consequences on the immune system. Early emotionally traumatic years may manifest in poorer coping responses to stress in adulthood. Psychological factors, such as our coping strategies, have been shown to be as important as the characteristics of the stress itself, in determining the immunological consequences of stress and the outcome of disease. For example, coping strategies and psychological factors have been shown to be significant predictors of who dies from acute asthma, in addition to predicting the progression of viral infections, AIDS, cancer and heart disease. On a positive note is the evidence that some coping strategies can minimise the detrimental effects of stressful life events; that positive emotional states can enhance immunity (for all references see Watkins 1997), and that some people's poor coping strategies can be shifted into more helpful and health promoting ones.

Clinicians are urged to consider the potentially massive positive psycho-physiological impacts that can be achieved as a result of treatment encounters, and that the ANS is regarded as a major efferent pathway linking mind and body.

REFERENCES AND FURTHER READING

Camilleri M 1997 Autonomic regulation of gastrointestinal motility. In: Low P A (ed) Clinical Autonomic Disorders. Lippincott-Raven, Philiadelphia 135–145

Chaitow L 2000 Fibromyalgia Syndrome. A Practitioners guide to treatment. Churchill Livingstone, Edinburgh

Damasio AR 1995 Descartes' Error: Emotion, reason and the human brain. Picador, London

Damasio AR 2000 The feeling of what happens. Body, emotion and the making of consciousness. Vintage, London

Ebner M 1975 Connective Tissue Massage, Theory and Therapeutic application. R E Kreiger, New York

Gifford LS 1998 The mature organism model. In: Gifford LS (ed) Topical Issues in Pain 1. Whiplash—science and management. Fear-avoidance beliefs and behaviour. CNS Press, Falmouth 45–56

Gifford LS 1998a Central mechanisms. In: Gifford LS (ed) Topical Issues in Pain 1. Whiplash—science and management. Fear-avoidance beliefs and behaviour. CNS Press, Falmouth 67–80

Gifford LS 1998b Output mechanisms. In: Gifford LS (ed) Topical Issues in Pain 1. Whiplash—science and management. Fear-avoidance beliefs and behaviour. CNS Press, Falmouth 81–91

Gifford LS (ed) 2002 Topical Issues in Pain 4. Placebo. Muscles and Pain. Pain Management. CNS Press, Falmouth

Gifford J, Gifford LS 1988 Connective tissue massage. In: Wells PE, Frampton V, Bowsher D (eds) Pain Management by Physiotherapy. Butterworth Heinemann, Oxford 213–227

Grieve G P 1994 The autonomic nervous system in vertebral pain syndromes. In: Boyling JD, Palastanga N (eds) Grieve's Modern Manual Therapy. Churchill Livingstone, Edinburgh 293–308

Harati Y, Machkhas H 1997 Spinal cord and peripheral nervous system. In: Low PA (ed) Clinical Autonomic Disorders 2nd edn. Lippincott-Raven, Philadelphia 28

Head H 1893 On disturbances of sensation with especial reference to the pain of visceral disease. Brain 16: 1–132

Janig W, Habler H-J 1995 Visceral-autonomic integration. In: Gebhart GF (ed) Visceral Pain. Progress in Pain Research and Management Vol 5. IASP Press, Seattle 311–348

Janig W, Habler H-J 1999 Organization of the autonomic nervous system: structure and function. In: Appenzeller O (ed) Handbook of Clinical Neurology Vol 74 (30): The Autonomic Nervous System. Part 1. Normal Functions. Elsevier, Amsterdam 1–52

LeDoux J 1998 The Emotional Brain. The mysterious underpinnings of emotional life. Weidenfeld & Nicolson, London

Levine JD, Reichling DB 1999 Peripheral mechanisms of inflammatory pain. In: Wall PD, Melzack R (eds) Textbook of Pain 4th edn. Churchill Livingstone, Edinburgh 59–84

Luedecke U 1969 History, basis and technique of connective tissue massage. Australian Journal of Physiotherapy 15(4): 141–148

Mackenzie J 1909 Symptoms and their Interpretation. Shaw and Sons, London

Martin P 1997 The Sickening Mind. Brain, behaviour, immunity and disease. Harper Collins, London

Meyers GE 1986 William James: His life and thought. Yale University Press, New Haven, Connecticut

Milner P, Lincoln J, Burnstock G 1999 The neurochemical organisation of the autonomic nervous system. In: Appenzeller O (ed) Handbook of Clinical Neurology Vol 74 (30): The Autonomic Nervous System. Part 1. Normal Functions. Elsevier, Amsterdam 87–133

Pick JP (1970) The Autonomic Nervous System: Morphological, Comparative, Clinical and Surgical Aspects. Lippencott. Philadelphia

Pennisi E 1997 Tracing molecules that make the brain-body connection. Science 275: 930–931

Ritter S, Ritter R C, Barnes C D (eds) 1992 Neuroanatomy and Physiology of Abdominal Vagal Afferents. CRC Press, Boca Raton, Fla.

Sapolsky R M 1994 Why Zebras don't get ulcers. A guide to stress, stress-related diseases, and coping. Freeman, New York

Selye H 1978 The Stress of Life. McGraw Hill, New York

Selye H, Tuchweber B 1976 Stress in relation to aging and disease. In: Everitt A, Burgess J (eds) Hypothalamus, Pituitary and Aging. Charles C Thomas, Springfield

Sternberg EM, Gold PW 1997 The mind-body interaction in disease. Scientific American Special Issue: Mysteries of the Mind June: 8–15

Thacker MA 1998 Whiplash—is there a lesion? In: Gifford LS (ed) Topical Issues in Pain 1. Whiplash—science and management. Fear-avoidance beliefs and behaviour. CNS Press, Falmouth 27–43

Watkins A (ed) 1997 Mind-body Medicine. A clinicians guide to psychoneuro-immunology. Churchill Livingstone, Edinburgh

Watkins A 1997 Mind-body pathways. In: Watkins A (ed) Mind-body Medicine. A clinicians guide to psychoneuroimmunology. Churchill Livingstone, Edinburgh 1–25

Watkins LR, Maier SF, Goehler LE 1995 Immune activation: the role of pro-inflammatory cytokines in inflammation, illness responses and pathological pain states. Pain 63: 289–302

Wesselmann U 1999 Pain of pelvic origin (urological and gynecological). In: Max M (ed) Pain 1999—an updated review. Refresher course syllabus. IASP Press, Seattle 47–58

Wesselmann U 2000 Urogenital pain syndromes in men and women. In: Devor M, Rowbotham MC, Wiesenfeld-Hallin Z (eds) Proceedings of the 9th World Congress on Pain. Progress in Pain Research and Management, Vol 16 IASP Press, Seattle 551–566

Westmoreland BF, Benarroch EE, Daube JR et al 1994 Medical Neurosciences. Little Brown, Boston

Williams PL, et al (eds) 1995 Gray's Anatomy 38th edn. Churchill Livingstone, Edinburgh

2

Complex regional pain syndrome: Part 1

LOUIS GIFFORD AND MICK THACKER

Introduction

This section of *Topical Issues in Pain 3* is devoted to conditions that have been largely attributed to pathobiology of the sympathetic nervous system. The previous chapter overviewed the anatomy and basic physiology of the autonomic nervous system. This chapter discusses the cluster of presentations that are classified under the umbrella term complex regional pain syndrome. The chapter describes and discusses their features and some aspects of their mechanisms and manifestations that may be of interest to physiotherapists seeking a broader understanding of the complex multifactorial underpinnings. The following two chapters discuss the pathobiology relating to the known *pain* mechanisms involved in CRPS.

Why is it that some people develop incredibly complex symptom presentations, often after relatively little in the way of injury? Remarkable cases where minor traumas quickly develop dramatic presentations—a simple bang on the elbow is followed by swelling of the hand, marked loss of joint range of motion and intense pain over the whole forearm that soon becomes resistant to all attempts to relieve the pain and which can then develop into an ongoing and devastating problem—are part of the experience of most physiotherapists. Cases of patients who present with quite long term pain and disability that includes observations and/or complaints by the patient of feelings of swelling, temperature changes, blotchy skin, altered sweating, poor skin health etc., are not uncommon and are often attributed to 'sympathetic' mechanisms. Is this true? What do we know about the role of the sympathetic nervous system in producing these states?

Further, can these sometimes awful presentations be prevented from happening in the first place, and once they are established how should we be thinking about their management?

This chapter, and the next two, explores and reviews postulated and known mechanisms relating to pain states where the sympathetic nervous system has been assumed to have a significant role.

It seems logical to assume that the autonomic nervous system, and hence the SNS, has to be involved in some way in all injuries, pathologies and pain states. The SNS, under normal conditions, has been shown to respond to nociceptive activity and to the presence of pain (see previous chapter and also reviews by Vallbo et al 1979, Wallin & Elam 1997). The reasoning is that since tissue damaging events represent a threat to the system's homeostasis and survival, the SNS, whose prime role is to engage defensive mechanisms, is likely to play a role in activating and co-ordinating the body's responses to restore or maintain homeostasis. Unfortunately, this isn't how the bulk of the literature on the role of the sympathetic nervous system in pain states following pathology or injury appears to view the situation.

An important point is that in normal circumstances, while the SNS *responds* to pain, its activity does not significantly excite sensory neurones and *cause* pain. Thus, the 'adaptive' role of sympathetic activity in the presence of pain is focused more on 'recovery physiology' rather than on the production of pain (Michaelis 2000).

Complex regional pain syndrome—new terminology to replace old

The role of the sympathetic nervous system in pain states has been a long held and reasonable assumption. It is based on the belief that sympathetic activity or hyperactivity is in some way involved in symptom generation. This belief is backed up by the clinical finding that sympathetic blocks, or destruction of sympathetic nerves when used in conditions diagnosed as having sympathetically maintained pain (SMP), like 'reflex sympathetic dystrophy' (RSD), are occasionally good at relieving pain as well as symptoms like oedema and sweating that are so often attributed to abnormal SNS behaviour. Further support comes from the finding that in some patients pain associated with neuropathy and RSD can be provoked by injection of adrenaline or noradrenaline or other 'adrenoreceptor agonists' (see Torebjork et al 1995, Wall 1995), whereas in normal people these hormones have no pain producing effect.

However, there is considerable argument surrounding the hypothesised role of the sympathetic system and also great difficulty in classifying patient presentations accurately. For example, many patients who fit into the RSD category do not respond at all to sympathetic blocking and a great many who do respond find that the relief is only temporary (see Chapter 4). Some patients may respond to a sympathetic block early on in the course of their problem, but not later, or vice versa (Torebjork et al 1995, Wall 1995). It seems that some patients can shift from having pain that may be dependent on sympathetic activity to having pain that is not. Some pain mechanisms appear to move and change over time, even though the presenting symptoms may appear stable.

For the past 10 years or so the golden nugget status that the sympathetic system has achieved and held on to has been subjected to quite a strong challenge that has resulted in a revised downward rating (see Chapters 3 & 4.)

In an attempt to clarify the nature of RSD and the role of the sympathetic nervous system in pain states a working party of world experts was set up following an International Association for the Study of Pain 'Special Consensus Workshop' held in Orlando, Florida USA in 1993 (Stanton-Hicks et al 1995). As an example of some of the challenges facing the group, the problems with the term RSD are representative: 'The term RSD is used imprecisely as it refers to changes in soft tissue which may or may not depend upon the sympathetic nervous system, may not be the consequence of a reflex, and may occur later in the disorder' (see Stanton-Hicks et al 1995, p 128). The goals set out in the workshop were to examine the terms RSD, causalgia, sympathetically maintained pain (SMP) and sympathetically independent pain (SIP) and to revise the classifications and definitions for better clinical utility.

One overriding theme was that the continued use of the term 'sympathetic' was unhelpful as it implied a pathological mechanism attributable to the sympathetic system that lacked conclusive evidence and which may have provided a barrier to the consideration of alternative mechanisms or a multiplicity of mechanisms acting in concert.

The group chose to use 'Complex Regional Pain Syndrome' (CRPS) as an overall term: *complex* to denote the varied clinical phenomena in addition to pain (see below); *regional,* since the distribution of symptoms and findings are so general, widespread and beyond the area of the original lesion—often being in the distal part of the extremities and rarely on the trunk and face, but having the potential to spread to other body areas; and *pain* since it was the cardinal symptom and being so disproportionate to the inciting event (Stanton-Hicks et al 1995, Boas 1996).

Within the CRPS designation are two subsets: Types I and II; both depend on the apparent cause and on the presentation—see Box 2.1. Type I corresponds to the 'old' RSD and Type II to 'causalgia.' Essentially the difference between the two is that Type I follows a tissue injury and Type II follows a frank nerve injury. A major departure as a result of this classification is the separation of the previously implied focus on sympathetic elements or mechanisms from the definitions. The result of this is the recognition that virtually any disorder, including CRPS, may have a component of sympathetically maintained pain alongside pains whose mechanisms are quite independent of the system, hence the terms sympathetically maintained pain (SMP) and sympathetically independent pain (SIP) (see Figs 2.1 and 2.2).

A major effect of this new classification is the focus on the presentation's history and the constellation of signs and symptoms, rather than on a presumed mechanism that seems to have unfairly overburdened the sympathetic system with responsibility and ignored other mechanisms that may be more relevant.

55

An important point for physiotherapy is that mechanistic approaches to pain syndromes like this are not necessarily helpful since they represent an interventionist biomedical paradigm whose object is to recognise a pathobiological mechanism, usually related to a pain mechanism, and then to *directly* alter the mechanism in some way. The recognition that pain is one thing but function and having a life are others too, does not seem to enter the therapeutic equation too easily. Even so, most physiotherapists like to feel comfortable with the problem they are dealing with and the belief here is that knowing about the current state of the art with regard to mechanisms is an important issue.

Box 2.1   Classification: complex regional pain syndrome (CRPS)

CRPS describes a variety of painful conditions that usually follow injury, occur regionally, have a distal predominance of abnormal findings, exceed in both magnitude and duration the expected clinical course of the inciting event, often result in significant impairment of motor function, and show variable progression over time.

CRPS Type I (RSD)
The syndrome follows an initiating noxious event.

1. Spontaneous pain or allodynia/hyperalgesia occurs beyond the territory of a single peripheral nerve(s) and is disproportionate to the inciting event.
2. There is or has been evidence of oedema, skin blood flow abnormality, or abnormal sudomotor activity, in the region of the pain since the inciting event.
3. This diagnosis is excluded by the existence of conditions that would otherwise account for the degree of pain and dysfunction

CRPS Type II (Causalgia)
This syndrome follows nerve injury. It is similar in all other respects to Type I.

1. Is a more regionally confined presentation about a joint (e.g. ankle, knee, wrist) or area (e.g. face, eye, penis), associated with a noxious event.
2. Spontaneous pain or allodynia/hyperalgesia is usually limited to the area involved but may spread variably distal or proximal to the area, not in the territory of a dermatomal or peripheral nerve distribution.
3. Intermittent and variable oedema, skin blood flow change, temperature change, abnormal sudomotor activity, and motor dysfunction, disproportionate to the inciting event, are present about the area involved.

Sympathetically maintained pain
Pain that is maintained by sympathetic efferent activity or neurochemical or circulating catecholamine action, as determined by pharmacological or sympathetic nerve blockade. SMP may be a feature of several types of pain disorder, and is not an essential component of any one condition. Conditions without any response to sympathetic block are, by contrast, designated as having sympathetic independent pain states (SIP).

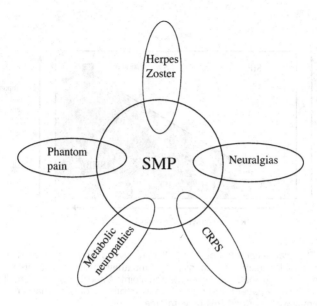

Fig. 2.1 Common pain conditions and the possible contribution of SMP to each.

Adapted from: Boas RA 1996 Complex regional pain syndromes: symptoms, signs, and differential diagnosis. In: Janig W, Stanton-Hicks M (eds) Reflex Sympathetic Dystrophy: a reappraisal. Progress in Pain Research and Management Vol. 6. IASP Press, Seattle 79–92

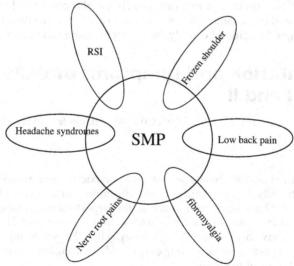

Fig. 2.2 As Figure 2.1 but including many common conditions seen by physiotherapists. Note that a 'sympathetic pain' component to these disorders is unproven at this stage.

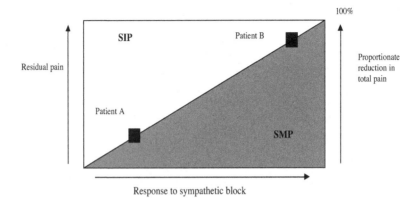

Fig. 2.3 The relative contribution that SMP may have to the overall pain. A: a person whose pain is predominantly unresponsive to sympathetic block. B: a patient with pain that is almost totally sympathetically maintained. Points A and B may represent different patients or the same patient at different times. In other words mechanisms of pain generation may well alter and change with time.

Adapted from: Boas RA 1996 Complex regional pain syndromes: symptoms, signs, and differential diagnosis. In: Janig W, Stanton-Hicks M (eds) Reflex Sympathetic Dystrophy: a reappraisal. Progress in Pain Research and Management Vol. 6. IASP Press, Seattle 79–92

Boas (1996) notes that a CRPS category III was also considered for 'those difficult cases that contained pain and sensory changes, with either motor or tissue changes, but did not comply fully with the more classic forms.'

Presentation and symptoms of CRPS Types I and II

Main sources: (Baron et al 1996, Low et al 1996, Birklein & Handwerker 2001)

Onset

CRPS Type I is almost always preceded by a noxious event usually to the affected extremity. Such trauma may be quite minor, such as a simple knock or bruising. But bone fracture, operations like carpal tunnel release or fascial releases for Dupytren's contracture, shoulder trauma, myocardial infarction or even CVA have been noted. A key feature is that the symptoms are often way out of proportion to the inciting event and have a tendency to generalise to the distal parts of the limb.

CRPS Type II is always preceded by a partial injury of a peripheral nerve or its major branches.

Sensory symptoms include pain and loss of sensation

- Intense ongoing pain.
- Pain frequently starts up and continues for no apparent reason. The literature describes this type of pain as 'spontaneous pain.'
- Ongoing hypersensitivity of the skin to touch and hypersensitivity to movement—i.e. touch and movement-related hyperalgesia/allodynia.
- Skin hypersensitivity, described as 'brush evoked pain' in reality is severe allodynia said to affect one-third of patients and an even higher incidence in chronic stages (a hallmark of central sensitisation.)
- Hypersensitivity of the skin to cold (cold allodynia). Found to be more frequent in CRPS Type II (60%, compared to 30% in CRPS Type I.)
- Pain quality is variable, often aching, burning, pricking or shooting in character and usually deep in the tissues.
- Sensory deficits tend to occur in a glove or stocking type distribution on the affected limb and often spread beyond the limb into the trunk.
- There is a sensory paradox. Areas where there is pain and hypersensitivity may also demonstrate decreased sensitivity/loss of sensation. For example patients are unable to feel the sharpness of a pin-prick in an area of skin that is painful when palpated. The suggestion is that a part of the problem has to be one of processing (a nervous system functional problem) rather than a structural one.
- The deep diffuse pain is often worse with the limb dependent by the side and better if it is raised up—the so called 'orthostatic' sign.
- Many patients find relief is also obtained by pressure around the affected area or proximal to the area. The use of the so-called 'ischaemia test' to diagnose RSD/CRPS is of interest here, because ischaemia, caused by the application of a suprasystolic cuff around the affected hand or foot produces significant relief of patients' deep diffuse pain (see Baron et al 1996). According to these workers, a positive ischaemia test has a 'high prognostic value' for pain relief generated by sympatholytic interventions. The mechanism by which this relieves pain is uncertain; Baron et al (1996) feel that it is likely that the ischaemia, as a result of decreased vascular filling, causes a decrease in activity of small diameter deep somatic afferents. The impact of ischaemia on symptom *development* in CRPS is discussed later.

Motor symptoms

- Weakness, tremor, exaggerated tendon reflexes, 'dystonic' posturing and myoclonic jerks. Dystonic means abnormal tone, and myoclonic jerks are shock-like contractions of groups of muscles, of variable regularity synchrony and symmetry. In classic medical literature these jerks are usually attributed to CNS lesions.
- In the acute phase there may be muscle weakness—possibly explained by pain inhibition or fear of harm/pain as it is a giving way type of weakness.

- In chronic stages it is hypothesised that weakness may be due to impaired muscle nutrition or/as well as abnormalities of central processing. Fear of pain and loss of confidence should also be a consideration.
- Tremor, myoclonic jerks and dystonia are reported to be more common in CRPS Type II.
- Reduced range of motion—by joint effusion and pain in acute stages and by contraction and fibrosis in chronic stages. Again, fear of pain and/or damage may be an important consideration.
- About 45% have exaggerated tendon reflexes on the affected side. Yet no pyramidal tract signs—but good correlation to level of pain. Therefore there may be a pain facilitation of tendon reflexes.

Autonomic symptoms

- Distal limb oedema.
- Skin colour changes—red in the early stages, turning bluish later.
- Skin temperature differences from affected side to good side—usually about 1°C. The affected side is warmer in the acute stages and cooler in the more chronic.
- In 50% of patients with CRPS increased skin sweating changes can be observed in the affected limb.
- Some researchers report that sweating may be increased or decreased and that it occurs most commonly on the palmar surface of the hand or plantar surface of the foot (Blumberg et al 1994). It is also noted that patients report a strange reaction of the skin temperature to changes of environmental temperature. For example, the affected hand in comparison with the healthy hand cools too slowly or too quickly when exposed to cold. Abnormal responses of skin blood flow to warming or cooling compared to the non affected side have been demonstrated in patients with RSD (Blumberg et al 1994).

Trophic changes

- Trophic changes occur in more than 50% of cases. Within a few weeks of the initiating traumatic incident there may be increased hair and nail growth. Thus there is an upregulation of growth in the early stages—so called 'plus signs.'
- Later, a decrease in tissue growth is observed—'minus signs'—here there is decreased hair and nail growth and atrophy of the skin. Skin may become thin and glossy and in severe cases there may even be skin ulcers.
- Other trophic changes noted are: changes in the *texture* of the skin, nails and hair; the skin may become fibrotic; there may be alterations in subcutaneous tissues as well as in bone density (osteoporosis). Plain radiographs show a diffuse and spotty distal distribution of demineralisation of small bones with a periarticular dominance at the longer bones (Baron et al 1996). These changes may not occur for many months. However, changes in bone metabolism picked up by 'three phase bone scans' apparently appear quite early on in CRPS Type I. Intraossary

plasma extravasation has also been demonstrated, which lends support to those who view the condition as an inflammatory disorder.

- It is not clear whether trophic changes are responsible for joint stiffness and tendon shortening. Disuse and functional motor changes may also have a role to play.

Note that it can be difficult to diagnose CRPS from some of the above reactions in the acute stage as many are the symptoms of normal trauma. For example, oedema, skin temperature differences and pain are commonly observed. Birklein & Handwerker (2001) state that the best symptoms to use for early recognition are motor signs, trophic changes and increased sweating.

Diagnostic tools

- In research laboratories and specialist clinics some workers use skin temperature differences—by measuring the affected and non-affected limbs repeatedly over time and in a variety of room temperature settings.
- Increased sweating in both the acute and chronic stages of the disorder are measured using a sudorometer.
- X-rays can reveal 'spotty osteoporotic changes' within 4–8 weeks, but only in 40% of cases. There is some evidence for increased bone metabolism.
- MRI scans show that muscle and periarticular tissues may become oedematous and there is an increased permeability of blood vessels, but it is a good deal less dramatic than that seen in arthritis.
- Diagnostic blocks alone are not helpful to diagnose CRPS but they are the only method to date that can indicate the possibility of a sympathetic component to the pain (see Chapter 4).
- Ischaemia test noted above.

Stages of the disorder

For some time CRPS (RSD/causalgia) has been considered to pass through three distinct stages (Bonica 1990) as an accepted fact in the literature. The stages or phases that were described by Bonica are:

1. The acute stage, characterised by pain and vasomotor changes such as generalised oedema, warm skin and sweating changes in areas not affected by the preceding lesion. These symptoms may occur within hours or days of the preceding incident.
2. The 'dystrophic' stage at 3–6 months after onset, characterised by more marked pain and sensory dysfunction, continued evidence of vasomotor abnormalities and markedly increased trophic and motor changes. The skin tended to shift from warm to cold.
3. The 'atrophic' last stage, with a decrease in pain/sensory disturbance, but continued vasomotor disturbance and markedly increased motor and trophic changes. For example, atrophy of muscle and bone and contractures of joints. This stage is seen as permanent.

This concept has now been challenged seriously. Recently Bruehl et al (2002), using a cluster analysis technique to look for stages in the disorder as well as different subgroups, were unable to support the existence of sequential stages. Their conclusions pointed to the existence of three different sub-types of the disorder:

1. A relatively limited syndrome in which vasomotor signs predominate.
2. A relatively limited syndrome in which neuropathic pain/sensory abnormalities predominate.
3. A florid CRPS syndrome similar to descriptions of classic RSD.

Interestingly, in their discussion Bruehl et al (2002) noted that in this third subgroup, work on animals as well as humans was suggesting a significant contribution of disuse to the development of the CRPS changes. They listed allodynia, hyperalgesia, motor dysfunction and temperature/colour changes. The negative effects of immobility are discussed further in the next section.

The results of this analysis reveal how highly respected and prominent individuals in a specialist area may be publishing unsubstantiated or even inaccurate material. We may need to be more wary of trusted experts and always in mind to check the sources on which their information is provided. Sadly, a good deal of the clinical 'facts' physiotherapists rely on may come into the same category and are really due for serious scrutiny.

Some mechanistic perspectives on CRPS

Immobilisation and disuse

Physiotherapists who have worked in a fracture clinic will be familiar with the appearance of a patient's limb when it is freshly taken out of plaster. On removal of the cast the limb is invariably atrophied, often with abnormal hair growth; it may be significantly warm with the skin being blotchy in appearance; it is markedly stiff; and occasionally it is very painful to touch and move. It actually looks very much like classic 'RSD.' Fortunately, only relatively few cases are known to go on to have a *documented* case of RSD or CRPS. However, the clinical reality, which urgently needs quantifying, is that many of the stubborn conditions physiotherapists treat have often had significant periods of quite unjustified immobility or disuse imposed on them.

That the features of CRPS may relate to disuse has been noted and the effects of immobilisation on humans and rats has been investigated (see Butler et al 2000). For example, Ushida and Willis (1996) immobilised rat wrists in full flexion for 3–4 weeks, some with radius fractures and some without. The results showed an increase in mechanosensitivity (touch and movement allodynia) in both groups and central plastic changes in spinal cord dorsal horn cells that process sensory information from the immobilised areas. Even immobilisation of rat hindpaws for one week will increase levels of sensitivity to heat, cold and mechanical stimulation (Maves & Smith 1996).

Four week immobilisation of the wrist in 21 human volunteers (Butler et al 2000) showed:

- All subjects had a temperature difference compared to the non-immobilised side ranging from 0.5–2.7°C (10 were warmer and 11 cooler). In three of the subjects the difference persisted longer than two weeks.
- 16 subjects had decreased range of movement of the thumb, 12 had altered sensation to sensory testing, of whom 4 had summation to pinprick (an amplifying sensation, often termed 'hyperpathia,' with every pinprick), and another four had hyperalgesia to pin prick.
- Pain was present in seven of the subjects—burning in two and aching in five.
- 18 reported stiffness and 14 had symptoms and signs of a 'neglect-like state.'
- Six subjects had abnormal sweating, seven had skin, hair or nail changes, and one had abnormal swelling.
- There was great variability in sensitivity to different and changing temperatures—some subjects becoming more sensitive while others became less. For example, in some there was a decreased tolerance to cold, often producing cold pain on the immobilised side. In contrast, some (two-thirds) had pain at a higher temperature on the immobilised side, indicating a decreased sensitivity; seven of the subjects were found to be able to detect the sensation of warmth earlier on their immobilised side; while in five others their warmth detection threshold was raised significantly.
- Some of the above changes lasted many weeks, but most were back to normal by 4–5 weeks.

There are some important clinical messages:

- Immobilisation is not healthy, it is detrimental. Immobilisation of normal wrists, let alone an injured one, causes quite dramatic changes in sensory processing, physical function, and physiological processing that can take quite a long time to recover in some individuals. Recovery appears to need activity and movement for return to normal. It seems that normal sensitivity and tissue health is maintained by normal use, a vital consideration for all those who would promote immobility or rest as a significant element of their intervention. What seems clear is that immobilisation is not a good thing and quickly leads to marked and quite remarkable changes that are not compatible with normal function, or normal sensory or physiological processing.
- We need to understand that there is great variability between individuals—there does not seem to be any typical response pattern. In an evolutionary setting 'in the wild' (see Gifford's Chapter in Volume 4 of this series, Gifford 2002a), immobility is only a very short term option no matter what is wrong. It is unlikely that an adaptive, biologically useful response has evolved to combat longer term immobility. Immobility is simply not compatible with survival. As a result, immobility can perhaps be classified from the very beginning as maladaptive.
- The constellation of findings associated with immobilisation are very similar to many of those found in CRPS Type I. It is not difficult to envisage

that a combination of injury and immobilisation in certain vulnerable individuals could lead to a long term disruption of sensory, motor and local physiological homeostatic mechanisms typical of those found in the CRPS conditions.

- The findings of the studies discussed provides some useful and reassuring information that can be passed on to patients who have been immobilised and are concerned about what they feel and see as well as the slow rate of progress. For example, even normal non-injured individuals immobilised for four weeks can have changes in temperature and touch sensitivity (up or down), swelling, pain, changes in skin and nail health, and sweating changes that can take many weeks to return to normal after cast removal. For the patient it is very reassuring to know that this is normal.

Neurogenic inflammation

Since the time of Sudeck at the turn of the last century the symptoms associated with the conditions now classified as CRPS (formerly Sudeck's atrophy, RSD, causalgia etc.) have been similar to inflammation, i.e. swelling, redness, pain and impaired function.

An important perspective is to look upon early inflammation following tissue injury as an *adaptive* process. Inflammation, albeit a much maligned process, should really be seen as the response that not only provides a hostile environment for potential invaders and attackers but also sets the scene for subsequent healing processes to develop. Part of the healing process of course, is for inflammation to subside and to be followed by processes of regeneration, repair, and remodelling. If inflammation continues on too long, in effect outstaying its welcome, it can then be seen as maladaptive. The ongoing, unsupressed nature of CRPS signs and symptoms, including those that appear inflammatory in nature, are surely maladaptive and hence have a negative impact.

Although classic humoral inflammation has never been proved, there is now good evidence to suggest that various measurable inflammatory and immune reactions are occurring in CRPS (see Veldman 1999). There are also some workers in the field who have pointed out how much of what is observed in CRPS resembles neurogenic inflammation (Birklein & Handwerker 2001, Weber et al 2001).

Recall that neurogenic inflammation is the effect caused by the stimulation of unmyelinated primary afferents—the C fibre nociceptors. Classically the 'axon reflex' is described as leading to the triple response: redness, flare and wheal in the skin following scratching. This circulatory response is known to be due to the release of neuropeptides from C fibres in the tissues of the skin.

The important message is that C fibres have a secretory or 'efferent' function (see Raja et al 1999) as well as a sensory or 'afferent' function. The end terminals of C fibres contain vesicles of neuropeptides that can be released into the tissues. Neuropeptides are thought to have an important trophic function in the skin (Tanaka et al 1988, Raja et al 1999) in that they support the tissues and help maintain their health. Think of C fibres as chemically sampling the tissues they supply, scrutinising what they find, and then helpfully responding if something is amiss by secreting various neuropeptides. In this way the C fibres effectively 'look after' the tissues they innervate and thus support their needs in times of difficulty. Thus, injured tissues need neuropeptides to activate a healing response.

It is known that activated C fibres release the neuropeptides CGRP (calcitonin gene related peptide) and SP (substance P) from vesicles in their nerve endings. CGRP release stimulates local blood flow by causing vasodilation of arterioles, and SP induces oedema by stimulating plasma extravasation from venules. Even though it has long been thought that plasma proteins are released during plasma extravasation in healthy skin, recent experimental studies, using high intensity TENS or capsaicin (chilli peppers), to stimulate the axon reflex, now show this may not to be the case (see Weber et al 2001). However, similar stimulation of the axon reflex and neurogenic inflammation in some CRPS patients, shows a clear early and short lived increase in plasma protein levels (Weber et al 2001). These findings led the authors to speculate that the presence of plasma proteins following the axon reflex should be viewed as a pathological finding.

What is apparent is that the observed swelling and increased skin vasodilation found in the early stages of CRPS strongly resembles neurogenic inflammation. The suggestion here is that for some unknown reason, either larger amounts of neuropeptides than normal are released from C fibres and/or their subsequent inactivation is physiologically impaired in someway. One group of researchers (Tanaka et al 1988) have suggested that an abnormal release of neuropeptides may be responsible for inducing the trophic changes observed in CRPS. Hence, increased hair growth rate in skin overlying the sites of fractures. Backing the role of neuropeptides as trophic stimulants is the finding that they play an important role in bone remodeling after fractures, that skin thickens near scars and that healing of wounds is accelerated by the presence of neuropeptides from sensory nerve endings. Denervation on the other hand reduces thickness of the epidermis and skin becomes hypotrophic (see Weber et al 2001). In CRPS patients, Weber and colleagues (2001) observe that in the acute phase there is an increase in hair growth in the affected area but that in the later stages skin becomes atrophic.

Another spin on peripheral vascular effects and neurogenic inflammation which fits the generally observed increased skin circulation, temperature, and redness of early CRPS noted above, may relate to 'antidromically' triggered vasodilation (Serra et al 2001). The mechanism here involves impulses passing down small afferent sensory fibres from the CNS to the periphery, i.e. the 'wrong way' or antidromically, with the subsequent release of CGRP. In the experimental situation, if freshly cut sensory fibres of nerve roots are stimulated electrically to produce antidromic impulses the skin supplied by that nerve root, i.e. its dermatome, reddens. Also, microstimulation of nerve fascicles that project to the skin of the hand, at intensities that produce a noxious effect, will cause a warming of the skin.

These effects have been shown to be independent of the sympathetic nervous system, as it occurs even after sympathetic postganglionic blockade.

It seems that neurogenic inflammation may have two sources: one where the impulses originate in the periphery—hence the well known 'axon reflex'; and the other where impulses actually originate from the CNS. In CRPS Type I, where symptoms and signs are critically distal or out of the territory of the inciting tissue injury, it seems that central origins of these impulses are likely. Certainly Sluka (1995) has addressed the physiology of a central origin to neurogenic inflammation via a 'dorsal root reflex'. It seems feasible that increases in central sensitivity and spread of sensitivity to segments beyond those immediately connected to the original injured tissues could have repercussions for the generation of increased antidromic activity to fundamentally normal tissues.

Oxygen-derived free radicals, oxidative stress, and ischaemia

In animal models intra-arterial infusion of compounds that produce oxygen-derived free radicals (oxygen radical donors) have been shown to cause reactions very similar to those of CRPS—oedema, increased skin temperature, impaired function, and pain behaviour (van-der-Laan et al 1998). Free radicals are therefore pro-inflammatory and their excessive production may result in destruction of healthy tissues. The significance of this is that trauma, inflammation, ischaemia, and circulatory reperfusion after ischaemia all trigger the release of these free radicals and support the potential for further negative effects.

In an article discussing the inflammatory aspects of RSD Veldman (1999) notes that even though there may be an increased blood supply through the affected tissues, there may still be poor oxygen saturation in the tissues themselves due to an oxygen delivery impairment. There may be plenty of blood, highly saturated in oxygen, but the tissues just seem not to receive it, hence they become hypoxic and suffer the effects of 'oxidative stress.' This may include a rise in oxygen-derived free radicals with the consequences already noted.

The reason for poor oxygen delivery is either that the blood coming into the area is shunted directly from arteries to veins, bypassing the microcapillary bed, or that it is a result of impaired diffusion from capillaries to cells. According to Veldman (1999) the second explanation is the most likely since 'an inflammatory reaction causes swelling of the intimal layers of the small blood vessels and their basal membranes, and hence a physical barrier to diffusion' (note the discrepancy here with the discussion in Chapter 3). Examination of the muscle biopsies from chronic RSD sufferers have shown evidence of oxidative stress—a decrease of Type I fibres, atrophic fibres, thickening of the basal membrane layers of capillaries, swelling and vesiculation of mitochondria, blebbing of the sarcolemnal membrane and disintegration of myofibrils. Thus, inflammation causes changes that lead to poor oxygen delivery which in turn causes hypoxia with yet further inflammatory effects. Part of the effect may well be driven by toxic build up of oxygen-derived free radicals.

Veldman (1999) feels quite strongly that oxidative stress may be the cause of post exercise pain flare-ups so often reported by these patients. He noted that patients often state that at the start of physical therapy exercises complaints of pain are mild, but by the end of the session and in the following few hours pain levels rise in parallel with the signs of inflammation. He states, 'RSD patients are not unwilling to perform exercises but are unable to recover from exercise' (Veldman 1999). While this has to be seen as a reasonable tissue-based explanation, other explanations relying on the effects of central nervous system hypersensitivity and phenomena such as wind-up and altered or impaired gating effects must be considered too (see Chapters 3 & 4.)

Interestingly, Veldman's thinking is supported by promising results of some preliminary trials using anti-inflammatory treatments specifically targeting free radicals with drugs that 'scavenge' for them. Two drugs that are used are mannitol and dimethylsulfoxide (DMSO), but Vitamin C is also a well known free radical scavenger.

According to Veldman (1999) a recent placebo-controlled trial by Zollinger et al (1998) using Vitamin C early on for patients with Colles fracture showed a marked prophylactic effect for prevention of RSD! Apparently, the results demonstrated a reduced incidence of post-Colles fracture RSD from a rate of 22% to only 8%. Veldman (1999) enthusiastically noted that this was the first report 'proving that RSD can be prevented.' It would be interesting to know the patient numbers, but unfortunately, the Zollinger et al (1998) article is in Dutch! In the bigger picture, as part of a multidimensional package of management, it is quite easy to encourage any patient with any form of injury or inflammatory problem to increase their intake of Vitamin C and to tell them that it helps in preventing long term problems with recovery.

A point made by Veldman (1999) is of interest and provides a useful thought to connect with the section that follows. He notes that there are only two animal models which induce RSD-like symptoms, the most well known being chronic constriction of the sciatic nerve model, and the other is via arterial infusion of an oxygen radical donor as noted above. The interesting question Veldman (1999) raises is whether it is the nerve injury that produces the oxygen derived free radicals or the oxygen radicals that produce the nerve injury!

Lastly, a few findings suggest that some of the increases in mechano-sensitivity in CRPS/tissue inflammation may in part relate to circulatory stress. For example, iontophoresis of the vasoconstrictor agents angiotensin II and vasopressin (Drummond 1998) slightly enhances hyperalgesia in skin that has been irritated and inflamed by capsaicin. Occlusion of blood flow has a similar effect (Drummond et al 1996).

Temperature changes, impaired sympathetic function, and supersensitivity development

The reader may recall from the previous chapter that noxious stimulation of viscera and the consequent sensory afferent barrage caused a *change* in sympathetic activity resulting in increased skin sweating and increased skin circulation with a consequent temperature increase. This activity may be relevant to the mechanisms proposed for abnormal skin temperature observed in CRPS. It may also provide one possible pathway for the development of the condition following deeper tissue injury. It would be interesting to know whether noxious stimulation of deep muscles or joints produces a similar change in sympathetic activity.

According to Veldman et al (1993) within the first weeks of CRPS, skin temperature and sweating on the affected limb are increased in nearly all patients, with the exception of a very few 'primary cold' cases. For those patients with increased temperature, this suggests, that sympathetic activity is in fact *reduced*. *Increased* sympathetic activity to skin causes vasoconstiction and hence *less* circulation to the skin (but see last paragraph below). Increased sweating on the other hand, is due to an *increase* in sudomotor sympathetic activity to sweat glands. Since most patients present with increased temperature and increased sweating it is suggested that the impairment of sympathetic output function (down for one, up for the other) is most likely to be of central origins (Wasner et al 2001)—but may have been instigated by afferent sensory barrages from injury or disease to other, possibly deeper, tissues.

If the clinical picture was one of increased temperature with a *decrease* in sweating the most obvious explanation, biased to the sympathetic system, would be loss of SNS activity. This might be due to pre- or postganglionic fibre injury / neuropathy / dysfunction, or to more complex central inhibitory effects.

Later on in the condition, when the disorder becomes chronic, skin temperature of the affected limb is almost always reduced compared to the good side. Patients complain that their limbs feel constantly cold. Indeed, clinical experience suggests that this is commonly the case in many chronic pain patients who may not necessarily be diagnosed as having CRPS. Is it due to altered or impaired sympathetic activity, or should we view it as merely the most likely consequence of disuse related to pain and hypersensitivity? Biomedical research tends not to think like this and mostly argues the case for altered physiological mechanisms. What mechanisms could explain this change in presentation?

Oedema

Most early CRPS presentations combine a heat increase with oedema of the distal limb. Could it be that the oedema is partly responsible for the second phase cooling? Oedema may produce an increase in tissue pressure sufficient to overcome normal venous filling pressure, causing collapse of the vessel and hence a point whereby circulatory perfusion is prevented. Once superficial blood flow velocity decreases or stops surface skin temperature will adapt to the ambient temperature which is normally colder than the core temperature. Loss of superficial circulation like this could also explain the tendency for skin health to suffer and lesions to develop. Clinically, and normally when we have cold hands or feet, it takes only a few minutes of active limb work to increase the circulation to the point where our extremities are very warm.

Oedema is discussed further below.

Supersensitivity development

In the nervous system it is known that following a peripheral nerve injury where nerve cells are actually killed and degenerate, i.e. where there is a frank neuropathy, the central sensory cells that normally connect to these primary sensory fibres that are 'lost', can develop a 'supersensitivity' state. It seems that central nerve cells involved in sensory pathways need their normal peripheral inputs and if they lose them they increase their sensitivity in an attempt to try and restore them. It is as if they are desperately looking for the slightest sign that their former fellows may still be found and the relationship rekindled.

This process of 'supersensitivity' development may occur outside the nervous system too. For example, with relevance here, it is postulated that a 'supersensitising' process may occur in the blood vessels of the skin when they are subjected to a decrease, or 'loss' of normal sympathetic activity (Birklein & Handwerker 2001). This may be due to ongoing reduced activity in sympathetic vascular output (discussed above), or, due to actual die-off of sympathetic postganglionic fibres if there has been a frank nerve injury (Wakisaka et al 1991).

Decreased sympathetic activity to the skin vascular bed effectively means reduced levels of the catecholamine transmitter noradrenaline in them. It is postulated that if this goes on for long enough the smooth muscle in the vasculature starts to increase its sensitivity to noradrenaline, for example by up-regulating the number of adrenoreceptors (Drummond et al 1996), with the result that they go on to develop 'catecholamine supersensitivity'. The vessels now become hyper-reactive to adrenaline whether derived from the sympathetic nerve terminals or from the adrenal glands via the circulation itself, and hence shift their activity state from being predominantly one of vasodilation to vasoconstriction. Support for this reasonable model is still thin (Birklein & Handwerker 2001) and alternative models have been proposed. One is the development of supersensitivity of central neurones associated with the production of vasoconstriction—hence a shift towards hyperactivity of skin vasoconstrictor neurones. This obviously requires an intact peripheral sympathetic supply. Another relates to the finding that re-innervated vessels demonstrate increased responses to sympathetic discharge and also to circulating levels of noradrenaline and adrenaline (Janig 1993). A possibility here is that, in the early stages, increased temperature relates to loss of sympathetic neurones while, later, decreased temperature relates to the supersensitivity that accompanies reinnervation.

Before leaving this section, with its interesting and competing hypotheses that attempt to explain temperature, sweating and circulatory changes, it is worth noting that there is some research available demonstrating a vasodilatory effect of the SNS to the skin on the dorsum of the hand and foot (Bell 1983, Lundberg et al 1989, Janig 1991). This is in direct contrast to the conventional belief, outlined at the beginning of this section and in the last chapter, that the activity of the SNS on the skin vasculature always causes vasoconstriction. For CRPS, the circulatory innervation and control to the dorsum of the hand and foot are of obvious interest. One wonders whether the innervation of CRPS sufferers is anatomically and functionally different from normals.

What some of the mechanisms highlighted in this section illustrate, whatever the underlying causative pathobiology, is that a decrease or loss of sympathetic activity needs to be entertained in the understanding and development of CRPS. What is also illustrated is the shifting nature of the mechanisms, the possible plethora of mechanisms and the potential for a wide symptomatic presentation, all of which serve to make any targeted biomedical approach to the problem very difficult. Unfortunately, the stability myth of nearly all pain states is often held down by diagnostic labels like 'reflex sympathetic dystrophy' and 'sympathetically maintained pain' (see Chapter 4).

Circulatory effects: sympathetically generated oedema

Blumberg et al (1994) describe four fascinating case histories of patients who developed 'RSD' with significant oedema that was dramatically relieved by sympathetic blocking procedures. The article is well worth reviewing and contains some very convincing pictures of the patients' condition before and after management.

To whet your appetite, what is so fascinating is the history of each and the dramatic onset of symptoms. For example, in the first case, a 37 year old healthy male merely banged his left elbow doing housework, carried on, had a nap for two hours and then woke to find severe swelling of the left hand and loss of sensation. The swelling was reduced dramatically by guanethidine blocks. The second patient, a 50 year old male who had kidney dysfunction for which he was on regular dialysis, underwent surgery to remove a subperitoneal haematoma. After coming round from the operation he complained of pain in his left leg that over the next few days focused on his foot and was accompanied by a massive swelling of the whole leg, in particular his thigh. The lower leg and foot were not only swollen but developed blisters. Here again, guanethidine blocks significantly and progressively alleviated the swelling and helped the problem to resolve.

These authors, in attempting to explain the oedema in these patients, after ruling out clear cut circulatory impairment, myocardial dysfunction or renal impairment, go on to dismiss an inflammatory or a neurogenic mechanism and propose a model that embraces an abnormal sympathetic discharge affecting in particular the vasoconstriction of veins.

The proposed hypothesis can be summarised:

- A lesion generates a nociceptive barrage into the CNS that sensitises 'spinal circuits' (see Chapter 3).
- The result of this spinal circuit excitation is an abnormal discharge pattern of sympathetic vasoconstrictor fibres.
- The oedema is generated because of the biased effect of the vasoconstrictor activity to the venous/postcapillary side rather than the arterial/precapillary side. Blood can flow in but cannot get out, hence an increased 'filtration pressure' which forces fluid out of the circulation and into the tissues.
- Increased pressure within the oedematous tissues then excites and activates their nociceptive population producing an afferent barrage that further maintains the sympathetic vasoconstrictor tone.

Whether vasoconstriction biased to the post-capillary side of the vascular bed is possible is discussed. Two things are proposed to support their hypothesis. First, that each section of the vascular bed is innervated separately by postganglionic neurones and therefore provides the potential for independent regulation of the calibre of pre- and postcapillary vessels. Second, pre- and postcapillary vessels react differently to the same activity in postganglionic vasoconstrictor neurones, the predominant action being biased towards the venous side.

A key element of the management paradigm is that it requires the existence of a vicious circle which can be interrupted in some way. Blocking the sympathetic side of the circle produced dramatic results. Vicious circles, if they are well founded, also leave open other therapeutic options; for example, could similar results be obtained by blocking the afferent traffic in nerves from the area affected? Since a peripheral nerve block prevents both afferent and efferent (hence sympathetic) activity it is feasible that this might be another approach.

Further, anything that could reduce the impact of afferent traffic or the potential for ongoing central sensitisation may be appropriate. Thus any form of therapy that reduces nociception or reduces the psychological impact of pain may be of some help. In a sense this is a simple plea for the possibility of multiple management strategies used 'in parallel' (Gifford 2002). This includes at one end of a spectrum cognitive-behavioural strategies and normal movement approaches and at the other the careful use of any active or passive input to help reduce the impact of nociceptive activity. Clearly, physiotherapists have a wide variety of skills and techniques to offer.

Unhealthy target tissues: a source of nociceptive input

This chapter needs now to hand on to the next two that take a closer look at the role of the sympathetic nervous system in pain. A final point before doing so is that associations between output systems and the input systems linked to pain may be quite indirect. Sympathetic or autonomic activity has the capacity to change the tissues that it innervates—for example a significant part of the discussion above relates to competing hypotheses focused on changes in circulatory perfusion. Thus, it seems quite feasible that altered sympathetic activity, especially if it is functionally disturbed in some way and is persistent (i.e. maladaptive), can lead to detrimental effects and impairments in the tissues it regulates and fosters. Long-term altered circulation, hence altered interstitial pressures and altered nutrition, oxygenation and clearance, is an example that cannot be compatible with positive tissue health. Nociceptive detection or 'sampling' systems may pass this information into the central nervous system with the potential to set up central sensitivity changes and hence pain states that may contain complex and multifaceted vicious circles.

REFERENCES

Baron R, Blumberg H, Janig W 1996 Clinical characteristics of patients with complex regional pain syndrome in Germany with special emphasis on vasomotor function. In: Janig W, Stanton-Hicks M (eds) Reflex Sympathetic Dystrophy: A reappraisal. IASP Press, Seattle 25–48

Birklein F, Handwerker HO 2001 Complex regional pain syndrome: how to resolve the complexity? Pain 94: 1–6

Blumberg H, Hoffmann U, Mohadjer M et al 1994 Clinical phenomenology and mechanisms of reflex sympathetic dystrophy: Emphasis on edema. In: Gebhart GF, Hammond DL, Jensen TS (eds) Proceedings of the 7th World Congress on Pain, Progress in Pain Research and Management. IASP press, Seattle 455–481

Boas R A 1996 Complex regional pain syndromes: symptoms, signs, and differential diagnosis. In: Janig W, Stanton-Hicks M (eds) Reflex Sympathetic Dystrophy: A Reappraisal. Progress in Pain Research and Management, Vol 6. IASP Press, Seattle 79–92

Bonica JJ 1990 Causalgia and other reflex sympathetic dystrophies. In: Bonica JJ (ed) Management of pain 2nd edition. Lea and Feibiger, Philadelphia, PA 220–243

Bruehl S, Harden RN, Galer BS et al 2002 Complex regional pain syndrome: are there distinct subtypes and sequential stages of the syndrome? Pain 95: 119–124

Butler SH, Nyman M, Gordh T 2000 Immobility in volunteers transiently produces signs and symptoms of complex regional pain syndrome. In: Devor M, Rowbotham MC, Wiesenfeld-Hallin Z (eds) Proceedings of the 9th World Congress on Pain, Progress in Pain Research and Management, Vol 16. IASP Press, Seattle 657–660

Drummond PD 1998 The effect of noradrenaline, angiotensin II and vasopressin on blood flow and sensitivity to heat in capsaicin-treated skin. Clinical Autonomic Response 8: 87–93

Drummond PD, Skipworth S, Finch PM 1996 Alpha (1) adrenoreceptors in normal and hyperalgesic human skin. Clinical Science 91: 73–77

Gifford LS 2002 Perspectives on the biopsychosocial model part 2: The shopping basket approach. In Touch, The Journal of the Organisation of Chartered Physiotherapists in Private Practice, Spring issue No 99

Gifford LS 2002a An Introduction to evolutionary reasoning: Diet, discs and the placebo. In: Gifford LS (ed) Topical Issues in Pain 4. Placebo and nocebo. Muscles and pain. Pain management. CNS Press, Falmouth

Janig W 1993 Pain and the autonomic nervous system : pathophysiological mechanisms. In: Bannister R, Mathias CJ (eds) Autonomic Failure, 3rd edn. Oxford University Press, Oxford

Low PA, Wilson PR, Sandroni P et al 1996 Clinical characteristics of patients with reflex sympathetic dystrophy (sympathetically maintained pain) in the USA. In: Janig W, Stanton-Hicks M (eds) Reflex Sympathetic Dystrophy: A reappraisal. IASP Press, Seattle 49–66

Maves TJ, Smith B 1996 Pain behaviours and sensory alterations following immobilization of the rat hindpaw. Abstracts: 8th World Congress in Pain. IASP Press, Seattle 118

Michaelis M 2000 Coupling of sympathetic and somatosensory neurons following nerve injury: Mechanisms and potential significance for the generation of pain. In: Devor M, Rowbotham MC, Wiesenfeld-Hallin Z (eds) Proceedings of the 9th World Congress on Pain, Progress in Pain Research and Management, Vol 16. IASP Press, Seattle 645–656

Raja S N, Meyer RA, Ringkamp M et al 1999 Peripheral mechanisms of nociception. In: Wall PD, Melzack R (eds) Textbook of Pain 4th edn. Churchill Livingstone, Edinburgh 11–57

Serra J, Ochoa J, Campero M 2001 Human studies of primary nociceptors in neuropathic pain. In: Hansson PT, Fields H, Hill RG et al (eds) Neuropathic Pain: Pathophysiology and Treatment, Progress in Pain Research and Management Vol 21. IASP Press, Seattle 63–83

Sluka KA, Willis WD, Westlund KN 1995 The role of dorsal root reflexes in neurogenic inflammation. Pain Forum 4 (3): 141–149

Stanton-Hicks M, Janig W, Hassenbusch S et al 1995 Reflex sympathetic dystrophy: changing concepts and taxonomy. Pain 63: 127–133

Tanaka T, Danno K, Ikai K et al 1988 Effects of substance P and substance K on the growth of cultured keratinocytes. Journal of Investigations in Dermatology 90: 399–401

Torebjork E, Wahren L, Wallin G et al 1995 Noradrenaline-evoked pain in neuralgia. Pain 63: 11–20

Ushida T, Willis WD 1996 Effect of contracture-induced pain in rat: Electrophysiological and behavioural study. Abstracts: 8th World Congress in Pain. IASP Press, Seattle 6

Vallbo A, Hagbarth K-E, Torebjork HE et al 1979 Somatosensory, pro–rioceptive and sympathetic activity in human peripheral nerves. Physiological Review 59: 919-957

van-der-Laan L, Kapitein P, Verhofstad A et al 1998 Clinical signs and symptoms of acute reflex sympathetic dystrophy in one hindlimb of the rat, induced by infusion of a free-radical donor. Acta Orthopaedica Belgium 64: 210–217

Veldman PHJM 1999 Inflammatory aspects of RSD. In: Max M (ed) Pain 1999—an updated review. Refresher course syllabus. IASP Press, Seattle 343–345

Veldman PHJM, Reynen HM, Arntz IE et al 1993 Signs and symptoms of reflex sympathetic dystrophy: prospective study of 829 patients. Lancet 342: 1012–1016

Wakisaka S, Kajander KC, Bennett GJ 1991 Abnormal skin temperature and abnormal sympathetic vasomotor innervation in an experimental painful peripheral neuropathy. Pain 46: 299–313

Wall PD 1995 Noradrenaline-evoked pain in neuralgia. Pain 63: 1–2

Wallin BG, Elam M 1997 Cutaneous sympathetic nerve activity in humans. In: Morris JL, Gibbins IL (eds) Autonomic innervation of the skin. Harwood Academic, Amsterdam 111–132

Wasner G, Schattschneider J, Heckmann K et al 2001 Vascular abnormalities in reflex sympathetic dystropohy (CRPS I): mechanisms and diagnostic value. Brain 124 (Pt 3): 587–599

Weber M, Birklein F, Neundorfer B et al 2001 Facilitated neurogenic inflammation in complex regional pain syndrome. Pain 91: 251–257

Zollinger PE, Tuinebreijer WE, Kreis RW, Breederveld RS 1998 Lagere incidentie sympathische reflex dystrofie bij polsfracturen na profylactische toediening van vitamine C. In: Van Mourik J B (ed) Posttraumatisch dystrofie. Gorssel: Symposium-commissie Chirurgie Nederland: 52–58

3

Complex regional pain syndrome: Part 2

MICK THACKER AND LOUIS GIFFORD

Introduction

Complex regional pain syndrome (CRPS) is a widely diagnosed yet poorly understood condition. It affects people of all ages and straddles all the major specialties of medicine (Janig 1996). The aetiology and pathology of CRPS remains unclear. There is continued debate over the precise role of the sympathetic nervous system in the generation and maintenance of the condition.

Most recent literature supports claims that CRPS is a pain state, a neurological disease, and an immune disorder. The major focus at the present time is on specific changes within the neuro-immune system at the cellular/molecular level. Older literature tends to suggest orthopaedic origins (Schwartzman & McLelland 1987). Despite a massive amount of research, the condition remains enigmatic and one that is very much open to confusion. Hopefully, the leading role that the International Association for the Study of Pain (IASP) has played in its attempts to clarify the situation will be beneficial for a more rounded understanding that is so needed (Stanton Hicks et al 1995, Janig 1996, this work is discussed Chapter 2). Even so, most work in this area remains tautologous and reductionist in its perspective.

Before the adoption of the 'CRPS' designation a great many different diagnostic labels were used that many clinicians will be familiar with. Box 3.1 lists some of the disorders that are traditionally associated with sympathetic dysfunction but which are now grouped under the umbrella term CRPS (see Chapter 2).

Box 3.1   CRPS synonyms in the literature

- Reflex sympathetic dystrophy
- Algodystrophy
- Disuse dystrophy
- Sudeck's atrophy
- Post traumatic dystrophy
- Traumatic vasospasm
- Shoulder-hand syndrome
- Peripheral acute troponeurosis

Recall from the previous chapter that the distinction between CRPS Type I and CRPS Type II is based on the precipitating event: CRPS Type I follows tissue trauma, CRPS Type II follows nerve injury and represents what was formerly described as 'Sudeck's atrophy.'

The term 'reflex sympathetic dystrophy' (RSD)

It is now the accepted convention to refer to the condition known as reflex sympathetic dystrophy (RSD) as complex regional pain syndrome Type I (CRPS-I). The current IASP definition is reproduced in Table 2.1 in the previous chapter.

Renaming from the old term was prompted by the confusion that it produced. Stanton Hicks et al (1995) stated that the term Reflex Sympathetic Dystrophy was used so indiscriminately and that it was no longer clear as to what it meant. These authors highlighted that the changes seen in the condition 'may or may not be the consequence of a reflex' and that there was a growing amount of evidence reporting no alteration in sympathetic nervous system output/reflexogenic discharge in individuals suffering this condition (Campbell et al 1992, Roberts 1986). They also felt that correct management should prevent the condition becoming dystrophic. The consensus from Stanton Hicks et al (1995) was that most of the dystrophic changes seen in this type of patient were probably due to pain related disuse rather than pathological processes.

More recently the new definition (see Chapter 2) has been criticised and it appears that the diagnosis of this condition is still fraught with difficulties (Galer et al 1998). A cynical (*clinical*) view might be that valuable time is wasted by trying to reach a consensus on what CRPS-I really is and not spent on the management of patients! The view proposed here is that a better understanding of the known, or hypothesised, underlying mechanisms will ultimately facilitate better management strategies and more broad based, multifactorial thinking.

Models for reasoning

In the early 1990s Wilfred Janig (Janig 1990, 1992), a leading authority on CRPS and the biology of the sympathetic nervous system, suggested that a new paradigm was needed to better understand the condition. He stated that any model that warranted widespread acceptance would have to have the ability to include changes within not only the sensory and sympathetic systems but also the motor and neuroendocrine systems.

In the first volume of this series Louis Gifford wrote four chapters that overviewed the known mechanisms of pain as well as reviewing some of the limitations of mechanistic ways of thinking (Gifford 1998, 1998a,b,c). He made a call for a more integrative approach to the understanding of all pain problems (Gifford 1998). In order to do this he proposed the use of his Mature Organism Model (MOM) as an educational tool to help both patients and clinicians adopt a far broader perspective than the current biomedical and pathologically based ways of thinking and reasoning pain.

This account reviews the literature in an attempt to identify and bring together many current thoughts on the CRPS conditions. The aim is to consider the 'disease' or syndrome within a wider context. In order to do this the material available has been integrated into the framework of the Mature Organism Model (MOM) (Gifford 1998). Whilst not aimed specifically at CRPS, this model may have the sort of broad validity required by Janig (1990, 1992).

The MOM offers an operative paradigm describing the continuous and dynamic biological processes and interactions involved in sustaining life. There are three main elements involved: first, those concerned with the sensory systems or what Gifford terms 'sampling' or 'input' systems; secondly, those systems concerned with the processing, 'scrutinising' or assessing of gathered information—for example the central nervous system; and thirdly, those systems concerned with action, 'output' or 'responding', hence motor/behavioural, sympathetic/autonomic, neuroendocrine and neuroimmune systems. The model places a shared and balanced emphasis on the physiological, psychological and behavioural aspects and their dynamic integration. Hence, body affects mind, mind analyses and affects body; body affects CNS, CNS analyses and affects body; environment affects CNS and mind; CNS and mind influence body and environment, and so on. Like the biopsychosocial model, the MOM approaches injury, disease and pain as multidimensional and multilevel phenomena that can impact all levels. Thus all pain, whether acute or chronic impacts all components of the model—the sampling, the scrutinising, and the output, and as such all have the potential to become impaired or dysfunctional in some way. It is as fair to consider the impact of impaired or dysfunctional physiological activity in damaged tissues and nociceptors as it is to consider along side this impaired or unhelpful beliefs, attributes and behaviours in an individual with a pain complaint (see Chapters 6 and 8). The reader is advised to consult the original material (Gifford 1998, 1998a,b,c).

CRPS mechanisms relating to 'sampling' systems

The MOM proposes that the peripheral sensory nervous system continually 'samples' its target tissues/environment and may then report on its findings to the CNS. Thus, quickly, via impulses or more slowly, via axoplasmic transport systems, sensory fibres can relay information on the health and condition of the structures they innervate to the CNS for scrutiny. It is also worth noting that many sensory fibres, notably C fibres, are known to have a trophic role and relationship with their target tissues (see Chapter 2). Thus C fibres and the silent afferents too (see below) not only sample, but also scrutinise and respond to changes in their target tissues at this cellular level. Hence, nociceptors that detect damage or pathology in the tissues they supply may provide a direct 'local' frontline response in the form of peptide release as well as informing the CNS for its 'opinion' regarding possible action.

Key sensory fibres involved in tissue sampling are nociceptors—the Aδ and C 'afferent' fibres. Their role in the production/maintenance of symptoms in CRPS has been the focus of numerous research papers. Much work relates to changes in sensitivity when their axons have been injured, are degenerate, or have been severed.

Nerve damage, nerve irritation and neuropathic changes

Damage to peripheral nerves and their neurons causes a series of well documented changes (Devor & Seltzer 1999). Following injury the afferent fibres acquire novel and abnormal properties resulting in an altered, usually increased, afferent barrage to the central nervous system. This leads, in turn, to an alteration in the normal functioning of neurons found in the spinal cord including those in the intermediolateral horn, i.e. sympathetic preganglionic neurons. This is the basis for many of the proposed models of CRPS (see among others Bennett & Roberts 1996, Blumberg 1992, Janig 1996, Koltzenberg 1996, McMahon 1991).

Most of the literature focuses on the findings from animal models of nerve injury. A major finding of these intentionally produced nerve lesion studies is that the small Aδ and C fibres are reduced significantly in number both within the dorsal root ganglion and the dorsal horn (Lisney 1992, Bennett & Roberts 1996). This results in the loss of incoming electrical and trophic signals, which are thought essential to the maintenance of normal CNS functioning (Woolf 1992). The nervous system may respond to this 'loss' of input by massively increasing its sensitivity, a situation that has been termed 'denervation supersensitivity' (discussed in Chapter 2.)

Note that there are two mechanisms here which can cause the CNS to upregulate its processing sensitivity or 'gain'—one in response to increased afferent barrage from damaged neurones that have become electrically hyperexcitable, and one in response to a loss of normal inputs due to the death and hence loss, of sensory fibres.

It is found that damaged sensory neurones that fail to fully regenerate and reach their original targets (Lisney 1992, Woolf 1992) may continue to show hyperexcitability, perhaps indefinitely. Clearly this will have a 'knock on' effect on both the scrutinising and output activities of the nervous system. In this way, nerve injury sets up the potential for ongoing increased sensitivity of dorsal horn neurons as well as many other cells and pathways throughout the CNS (McMahon 1992, Woolf 1992).

What is clear, is that damage to peripheral nerves can have quite far reaching repercussions on the processing and output pathways of the CNS. This poses problems for 'conventional' targeted approaches and pain treatments. The more research reveals about pain mechanisms the more traditional approaches are being forced to consider multiple sources, factors and mechanisms in many pain conditions. Thus, biomedically, a focus on a single peripheral source of pain may be inadequate in CRPS or for that matter any injury that causes pain, particularly the longer it has been established.

In addition to the above changes, many damaged sensory fibres demonstrate spontaneous activity in the form of ectopic impulse discharges (see Devor & Seltzer 1999 for an in depth discussion of the processes underlying these phenomena.) This is a well known peripheral mechanism that is thought to account for the spontaneous pains unrelated to any movement or other stimulus often reported by patients with neuropathic pains.

Spontaneous activity from injured nerve fibre axons is likely to result in pain or symptoms in the tissue areas that the affected nerves normally innervate. Thus, ectopic impulses generated from nociceptive nerve fibres that normally innervate the calf muscle will be 'felt' as pain in that muscle. The warning for the clinician is that nerve fibre hyperexcitability can result in pains in tissues that may be relatively normal. What is abnormal is the activity of their sensory supply.

The processes outlined here appears to present a perfect model for the initiation of neural changes that could lead to the development of CRPS. However, it is important for the reader to appreciate that the above findings are the results of direct nerve damage in animal models. There is some evidence to suggest that these injuries do not resemble those that are sustained by individuals who develop CRPS (Lisney 1992). This point has received a lot of attention in the literature. There is however a consensus that *careful* extrapolation from animal models of underlying mechanisms for individual symptoms is acceptable (Bennett & Roberts 1996, Janig 1996, Koltzenberg 1996).

Generally, the clinical picture of CRPS has been used by many as a reliable indicator of neural damage. Particular attention has focused on the presence of hyperalgesia to mechanical stimuli. Drummond et al (1996) biopsied skin from areas of hyperalgesia in subjects with established CRPS in an attempt to identify peripheral neural pathology. They compared these skin samples with those taken from areas of normal sensation in the same subjects. They found an increased number of 'nerve tangles' in the hyperalgesic region compared with the control areas but the differences did not reach statistical significance.

79

These rather weak findings for peripheral nerve abnormality appear to support the view of Lisney (1992) who concluded that hyperalgesia in CRPS is not likely to be as a result of direct changes in afferent fibres. He suggested a more central origin for these symptoms.

New experimental animal models have been developed that cause minimal direct axonal damage but rather promote an immune/inflammatory reaction in peripheral nerve trunks (Eliav et al 1999, Maves et al 1993). These models may prove to be more applicable to the study of the mechanisms relevant to CRPS Type I.

Electrical coupling

Undamaged normal afferent and efferent neurones show functional independence from adjacent fibres, that is, they are not stimulated by or cause the stimulation of their neighbours. Following nerve damage this situation can be altered with adjacent neurones demonstrating 'crossed excitation' (Devor & Seltzer 1999). Under such circumstances the firing of one neuron leads to the depolarisation of adjacent neurones to which it has newly made inappropriate contacts. Thus one explanation why normal movements might cause significant pain might be that mechanoreceptor or proprioceptor barrages mediated by Aβ nerve fibres with normal movement would be able to excite adjacent nociceptors that have acquired cross excitation capability. The normal and innocuous sensory signals effectively migrate into the pathways that process pain.

The nature of these contacts has been the source of widespread discussion in the literature. Early attention focused on the presence of false 'electrical' synapses known as ephapses (Doupe et al 1944, Granit & Skogland 1945). Lisney (1992) commented that these false synapses are only found in nerve end neuromas, but others have found them in regenerating nerves distal to the site of injury and in patches of demyelination (see, Devor & Seltzer 1999). However, so far, there is little evidence for this type of structural change in CRPS patients or the animal models that are used to reflect CRPS symptomology. Devor (1991) and McMahon (1991) have reported a scarcity of false synapses in animal models and have identified that when present, the coupling is between sensory fibres and does not involve the sympathetic fibres. Their presence in humans is unproven at the present time. However, there is a growing body of evidence to suggest that chemical coupling of sensory and efferent sympathetic fibres does exist (Devor 1991 & 1994, Koltzenberg 1996, Lisney 1992, McMahon 1991, Michaelis 2000).

Chemical coupling

Wall and Gutnik (1974, 1974a) were the first to demonstrate that damaged nerve fibres showed an increased sensitivity to adrenaline and noreadrenaline. Many developments of this early work have now appeared in the literature (Devor 1991, 1994, 1996, 1999; McMahon 1991, Michaelis 2000).

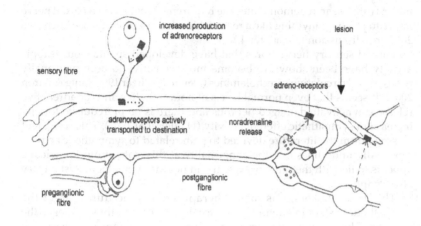

Fig. 3.1   The effect of nerve injury on adrenaline sensitivity. A nerve injury or lesion leads to an increase in adrenosensitivity. This is due to increased production and activation of adrenoreceptors.

Adapted from: Janig W, McLachlan, EM 1994 The role of modifications in noradrenergic peripheral pathways after nerve lesions in the generation of pain. In: Fields HL, Libeskind JC (eds) Pharmacological Approaches to the Treatment of Chronic Pain: new concepts and critical issues. Progress in Pain Research and Management Vol. 1. IASP Press, Seattle

It is important to note that damaged afferent nerve fibres show increased receptor expression for catecholamines, in particular, alpha-1 and alpha-2 adrenoreceptors (Devor 1996) (see Fig. 3.1). Thus, damaged sensory fibres change plastically by up-regulating (producing more) adrenoreceptors and activating refactory (dormant) adrenoreceptors. The result is an increase in the presence of active adrenoreceptors in the sensory fibre. No matter where the nerve is lesioned the adrenoreceptor increase may be far reaching. Active adrenoreceptors have been found on the cell bodies, axons, axon terminals, re-growing sprouts of damaged nerve fibres, and in nerve sprouts in neuromas. The end result is that the fibres become more sensitive to adrenaline and noradrenaline (see Coderre et al 1989). Devor (1996) stated that the aetiology of SMP in CRPS effectively boils down to adrenosensitivity on the sensory side as opposed to excessive output of adrenaline or noradrenaline on the (sympathetic) efferent side.

However, in CRPS Type I, there is no apparent or detectable nerve injury, which raises the question of how significant adrenosensitivity might arise here. Interestingly, there is modest evidence (discussed further later) to show that sensitised nerve endings in inflamed tissue can also become adrenosensitive (Levine et al 1986, Sato et al 1993, Drummond 1995). An important point is that there may not have to be a nerve injury for the development of adrenaline/noradrenaline chemosensitivity. Still, the vast majority of research demonstrates the requirement of at least a partial nerve injury to produce anything like a reasonable adrenosensitivity (see Michaelis 2000 and discussion in Chapter 4.)

Injured sensory nerve fibres that have developed spontaneous ectopic activity have been shown to become more sensitive to both neuronally released and circulating catecholamines (Devor & Seltzer 1999, Janig & Baron 2001). It seems that even normal levels of noradrenaline and/or adrenaline release can activate damaged neurons and there is no prerequisite for any increase in sympathetic efferent activity (Habler et al 1987). This consistent message from the literature devoted to pain related to sympathetic activity repeatedly underlines that the abnormality at this state of our knowledge appears to lie with the sensory system and not the sympathetic system (see also Chapter 4).

This is a vital point as many therapies and procedures target the sympathetic system in attempt to reduce its activity and thus influence the disorder. There is potential for a reasoning error if therapies are based on shaky evidence. Although there is little doubt that methods that decrease the amount of noradrenaline in the circulation and/or tissue (e.g. relaxation) can benefit the individual, the consensus of biomedical opinion (Janig 1996, Michaelis 2000) is against interventions that aim to inhibit the postganglionic fibres directly in order to alter sympathetic output, e.g. interferential currents.

The increased expression of alpha adrenoreceptors on the cell membranes of damaged afferent terminals and re-growing axons has already been discussed. Coderre et al (1989) demonstrated similar increases of adrenoreceptors in the cell membranes of dorsal horn and dorsal root ganglion (DRG) cells of rats. This increase followed significant afferent barrage activity from a neuroma following nerve injury. This is another example of neuroplastic change in this condition, and supports the concept that the pathology that underpins CRPS need not reside in the periphery where symptoms are felt.

Coderre et al (1989) concluded that the presence of such receptors, wherever they occur on sensory afferents, offer a ready answer as to how efferent sympathetic activity can cause firing of damaged afferents. It is important to reiterate that the receptors are sensitive to adrenaline and noradrenaline regardless of its source of origin. Therefore circulating adrenaline released into the blood stream (e.g. result of psychological stress) could, possibly, cause an increase in nociceptive barrage and hence pain.

This is important information for the clinician as many CRPS patients complain of increased pain during periods of emotional stress. For example tension generated by physiotherapy appointments could exacerbate pain, especially if there have been previous negative experiences.

McMahon (1991) has also proposed an indirect coupling of the sympathetics with the afferents. This involves the autoexcitation of the sympathetic efferents, with the subsequent release of prostaglandins, a known inflammatory and pain producing agent (this concept is discussed in further detail below).

Silent afferents

In addition to increased impulse discharge from 'normally active' nociceptors there appears to be a novel afferent barrage produced by a sub group of nociceptors that have received increasing attention in the literature. These sub-types are known to remain silent even when extreme physical or physiological conditions occur. Thus, even when stimulated at levels that are known to cause normal nociceptors to discharge they fail to fire. It is for this reason they are often referred to as 'silent' or 'sleeping' afferents/ nociceptors. It seems that they come into their own in the aftermath of tissue injury during the early inflammatory stages. In these conditions, probably stimulated by inflammatory agents, they 'awaken' and display increased excitability. (For a detailed account of the behaviour of these fibres see McMahon & Koltzenburg 1990, 1990a.) There is evidence that input from these silent afferents has a greater impact on CNS processing and sensitivity changes than that derived from activity in 'normal' nociceptors (Wall, personal communication). This may be significant in the development of CRPS and other chronic pain syndromes.

Is there a nerve injury in CRPS Type I?

The bulk of the discussion so far, on CRPS and SMP, is based on findings from animal models of neural damage and a subsequent increase in adrenosensitivity. As outlined in the previous chapter, the IASP definition of CRPS Type I requires that no history of relevant nerve injury has occurred, which makes the research discussed seem irrelevant to this condition. The definition also states that the diagnosis of CRPS is excluded by the existence of conditions that would otherwise account for the degree of pain and dysfunction. Problems arise here as better investigative screening and work-ups find lesions that would otherwise be missed—and hence challenge the classification of the disorder. For example it may be possible that many conditions designated CRPS Type I do in fact have nerve impairments or dysfunctions that are relevant, or could even be reclassified as neuropathies when scrutinised more closely. Thimineur and Saberski (1996) discuss this difficulty. They report three case studies of patients who were diagnosed as suffering CRPS Type I but were subsequently found to have nerve entrapments. Two of these individuals were reported to have a total resolution of symptoms following decompression of the entrapped nerve. Although impressive, no longer term follow ups were reported by these authors.

Thimineur and Saberski (1996) discuss the validity of the IASP definition of CRPS in light of their findings and suggest that oversights may occur if one accepts a diagnosis too readily. As anywhere, carefree labelling in patients exhibiting what in many cases are normal sequelae to injury, could lead to the patient receiving inappropriate (often protracted) management strategies. More detailed screening of patients may reveal alternative explanations for the patient's clinical presentation, and sometimes, the potential for more appropriate management. We must be aware that the overzealous diagnosis of RSD / CRPS has received criticism in the literature (Janig 1992).

CRPS mechanisms relating to the 'scrutinising' systems of the CNS

We now know, from the work of Wall, McMahon, Woolf and others, that pain generating mechanisms that have become established in the periphery can have significant impact on the processing mechanisms within the central nervous system.

The clinical presentation of CRPS has led to the implication of the CNS both in the production and maintenance of symptoms (McMahon 1992, Janig 1992,1993, Blumberg 1992). For example, clinicians frequently encounter patients demonstrating extreme, prolonged, and maladaptive hypersensitivity states. The mechanisms underlying the conditions of hyperalgesia and allodynia are known to involve CNS changes (McMahon 1992, Woolf 1992). Also, the extensive and regional nature of the symptoms strongly suggests CNS involvement. Changes within the CNS are thought to be implicated where pain spreads to affect an entire region following an isolated lesion. Current knowledge suggests that the best explanation for this remarkable phenomenon relates to the maladaptive expansion of dorsal horn cell receptive fields (see Woolf 1992).

Louis Gifford outlined the role of the central nervous system in the production and maintenance of pain in the first volume of this series (Gifford 1998b). Similar changes are thought to occur in CRPS patients. The two main processes known to operate under such circumstances are 'wind-up' and 'sensitisation.'

Central changes in sensitivity and excitability within the dorsal horn are known to result from ongoing afferent impulse barrages derived from sensory neurones that supply or come from the site of injury. The afferent barrage reaches the second order target neurons in the dorsal horn[1] and sets in motion a series of electro-chemical reactions that alters their excitability. Several processes are thought to occur in parallel (see Fig. 3.2A, B and C).

1. The electrical impulse discharge that arrives at the afferent fibre terminals causes the release of an excitatory amino acid neurotransmitter called glutamate (Fig. 3.2A). Glutamate crosses the synapse to the second order neurone where it acts on a specialised AMPA receptor. If enough glutamate is released it effectively causes, via the AMPA receptors, the depolarisation of the dorsal horn neurons with a subsequent influx of both calcium and sodium ions into the neurone. Glutamate release thus increases the excitability of the second order neurone.
2. Further/continuous afferent barrage also causes the release of another neurotransmitter, substance P, from the afferent sensory fibres (Fig. 3.2B). Substance P then crosses the synaptic cleft and acts on available 'neurokinin' receptors on the second order neurones. This results in a further influx of calcium and sodium ions into the second neurone as

well as stimulating the release of calcium from stores within the cell. Calcium ions are known to be key 'messengers' responsible for increased responsiveness and excitability of the second neuron. The result is that the cell becomes 'charged', raising its excitability and sensitivity still further (Woolf 1992, 1994).

3. If the discharge of the primary afferent continues the intracellular sodium and calcium ion concentrations of the second neurone reach a critical level which leads to the activation of a previously blocked receptor type, the NMDA, or N methyl D aspartate receptor (Fig. 3.2C). The activation of the NMDA receptor involves the removal of a bound magnesium ion within it. This is caused by a change in its configuration triggered by the intracellular increase in calcium noted above.

4. Following the removal of the magnesium ion the NMDA receptor can be activated by further/on-going release of glutamate. Like the AMPA receptor, this activated NMDA receptor causes the cell to increase its potential flow of ions, and hence its electrical reactivity. In this way the cell up-regulates its firing capability. Now the second cell not only has a population of AMPA receptors available, but is also joined by activated NMDA receptors on which the glutamate can act. The result of this effective 'increase' in receptors is an increase in the cells ability to respond and fire to arriving glutamate. The cell firing becomes amplified in both amplitude and duration. These electrochemical changes form the basis of both wind-up and sensitisation. (For an in depth account see Doubell et al 1999, Coderre et al 1993, McMahon et al 1993, Woolf & Thompson 1991.)

Wind-up is a relatively short lasting process that requires an ongoing afferent impulse volley into the cord. *Sensitisation* is a long lasting process thought to be synonymous with the process of long term potentiation (LTP). LTP is a process widely studied in the hippocampus of the brain in respect to memory and learning and which is known to have the ability to persist for extended periods of time (Coderre et al 1993; Rose 1992).

Later sequelae that may result from the impact of nociceptive activity on the dorsal horn include:

- The formation of novel synapses—for example, Aβ fibres that normally terminate and synapse in lamina III/IV and V of the dorsal horn may sprout and form synapses in the outer laminae where nociception is processed. Thus normal, innocuous, proprioceptive and sensory inputs from normal tissues may, via this novel route, enter the nociceptive system and be processed in terms of pain (see Doubell et al 1999).

- The death of inhibitory interneurones in the dorsal horn, so called amino acid 'excitotoxicity' (Dubner & Ruda 1992). Here, high levels of excitatory amino acid neurotransmitters (i.e. glutamate) may actually lead to cell death. It seems that inhibitory interneurones are most vulnerable here. The clinical impact is that the system has lost some of its normal control mechanisms over nociception. This type of knowledge helps give a far better explanation for pain that takes many hours to calm down or that builds up very easily and quickly.

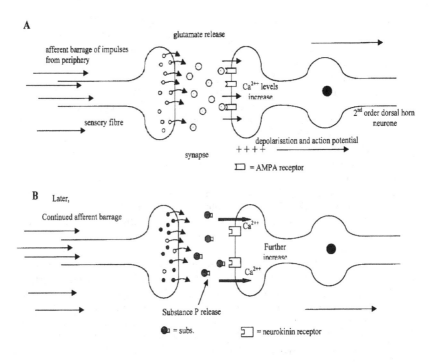

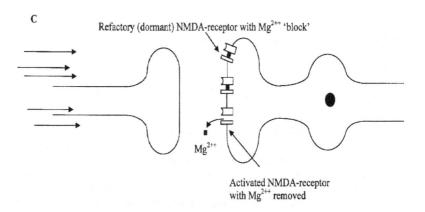

Fig. 3.2A, B, & C Some of the known synaptic events that occur in setting up sensitivity changes in the spinal cord dorsal horn.

Wind-up

Clinically, wind-up refers to the gradually increasing pain response that occurs when a given stimulus is repeated. For example, a CRPS patient may feel pain in the leg with ankle movement and with every repetition of the same movement the pain builds and builds to excruciating levels in a seemingly uncontrolled way.

Wind-up requires ongoing input into the system. This may be provided not only by repetitive stimuli, but also by the spontaneous generation of ongoing impulses from injury sites on peripheral nerve fibre axons as reviewed earlier, or even from relatively minor tissue injury sites. Whatever its origins, the ongoing input causes central changes similar to those described in the last section.

It seems that as the repetitive input is delivered to the CNS so the second order cells become more and more excitable and hence fire more and more easily. In animal models at least, if this afferent impulse activity is stopped or blocked the increased excitability generated in the secondary neurone diminishes and will rapidly return to a normal level. In a few patients it has been found that immediate and lasting relief occurs in response to procedures that block the afferent barrage (Wall 1995).

If this 'wind-up' scenario is the case for the highly sensitised CRPS patients it is little wonder that their attempts to get moving or do exercises are so easily beaten back by massive and long lasting increases in pain.

Concomitant tissue changes, such as neurogenic inflammation, alterations in circulation, local hypoxia, tissue deconditioning, oedema and tissue disuse, could all lead to an increase in peripheral sensitivity and afferent barrage further reinforcing the setting up and maintenance of central changes. This all suggests that our management strategies should carefully balance attempts to attend to and calm sources of ongoing input into the system with prevention of deconditioning. This means establishing progressive and paced early functioning. The emphasis here is on 'early' so as to avoid, as far as possible, the potential for maladaptive central changes becoming established. The cognitive-behavioural and self management approaches for the more established CRPS pain condition described by Suzanne Brook in Chapters 6 & 7 are important, as they allow time for gradual change and acceptance by the nervous system as well as the individual who is attached to it.

Sensitisation

Sensitisation differs from wind-up in that, once initiated, ongoing activity of the central neurons may continue *even in the absence of further afferent input*. Coderre et al (1993) describe two ways in which sensitisation may be initiated: the first is by continued low frequency input into the system: it can also be from a short lasting high intensity afferent burst into the CNS, a so-called 'neural scream' (Coderre et al 1993). This is of interest in the study of CRPS as the condition is often reported to have arisen from injuries that produce a short lasting but highly intense burst of nociceptive input. This certainly occurs when an intact nerve is cut during animal experimentation (Devor & Selzer 1999).

Clinically, established sensitivity is a major hurdle and may be significant reason why many ongoing problems just do not respond to pain relief therapies satisfactorily. This is probably the single most important reason to persuade us to move towards management models that embrace pain management and improved function as outlined here by Brook (Chapters 6 & 7) and in many chapters in the other Topical Issues in Pain volumes of this series.

Mind-body link to the impact of wind-up and central sensitisation

Since there are known descending excitatory and inhibitory pathways from brain to spinal cord dorsal horn (reviewed in Fields & Basbaum 1999), it seems plausible that changes in mental state, like feelings of wellbeing, mood, expectation, learning and attention may impact the injury related afferent barrage effect on the central plasticity state. It is certainly known that activity of dorsal horn nociceptive neurones can be modulated up or down depending on the context in which painful stimuli occur. Changing the focus of attention towards the stimuli that produce pain, or to the pain itself, will increase the responsiveness, and changing it away reduces it (reviewed in Petrovic & Ingvar 2002). Prolonged focus of attention on pain often occurs in patients who have significant levels of pain or who are highly concerned about it or cannot for whatever reason make sense of it. Continued interest in pain, via central facilitatory pathways and mechanisms, will surely reinforce the electrochemical effects on the central cells leading to long term sensitivity changes and even to the potential for central pain generation (see Gifford 1998b). Fields and Basbaum (1999) do raise the possibility that pain could even *originate* from the CNS given enough central facilitation of dorsal horn neurones associated with nociception. See also the opening chapter by Melzack in this volume.

With this type of understanding it can be seen that even relatively minor degrees of nociceptive activity in the presence of significant cognitive or affective turmoil could have a more profound effect than if conditions were more evenly balanced. Also, it seems quite feasible neuroplastically that according increased attention to a given sensation can actually cause it to create a larger neurological impact on the CNS than if it were given less credibility or ignored. After all, if you want to learn something you have to concentrate on it (Gifford 1998b). Implications for early management and prevention of chronic pain and its impact, are to provide effective reassurance as quickly as possible, provide effective pain relief, and for the individual to keep active and occupied. It seems that doing nothing for too long allows us to dwell on and hence better establish our symptoms. The combination of emotional turmoil, uncertainty and increased attention to symptoms may be significant factors worthy of respect and consideration.

Are we then at risk of complex and chronic pains developing from acute injuries or acute pain onsets that are accompanied by heightened stress or depression? There is some support for this reasoning in the literature.

Van Houdenhove et al (1992) proposed a biopsychosocial hypothesis for the etiopathognesis of reflex sympathetic dystrophy. They screened a group of patients suffering reflex sympathetic dystrophy for psychological disturbances. They found that at the time of the initiating injury the patients had experienced an 'existential loss,' either as a direct result of the injury or exacerbated by it. They proposed a model of how this loss could lead to ongoing psychological and physiological symptoms. This may be an important and unique piece of work. In particular, it attempts to assess the affect of injury in the context of both the tissues and the mind and it offers a hypothesis that the 'unfortunate' timing of an injury could lead to amplification of normal adaptive responses to a maladaptive level. It seems reasonable that an individual who is under pressure—be it psychological, physical or both—is in a state of 'vulnerability' or 'reduced capacity to cope', and therefore less able to deal psychologically, physically, and physiologically with any additional burdens that may occur.

The more positive side of the coin is that acute management strategies that help patients to reduce the impact of pain (intensity and emotional), and that put the pain in a less threatening context by reducing levels of anxiety and fear, could well prevent its central impact from becoming maladaptive and hence chronic. Even in the longer term pain sufferer these strategies may be helpful. If something can be deemed unimportant, less threatening, or of little consequence it usually gets ignored. If this can become established, then positive neuroplastic changes to processing pathways are likely to have occurred.

Higher centre dysfunction?

Janig (1992) suggested the potential for dysfunction in the limbic system and the brain stem in CRPS patients. Until recently this theory has remained largely untested.

Thimineur et al (1998) published the results of their clinical study of 145 patients with CRPS. They assessed CRPS patients, patients with other pain conditions, and normal patients, for signs of brain stem dysfunction, and found a high incidence of trigeminal hypoaesthesia and lower cranial nerve (nerves 11&12) dysfunction in the CRPS patients. This finding, along with high incidences of bilateral motor weaknesses, was used as supporting evidence for their hypothesis that a sub-population of CRPS patients have dysfunction of their brain stem. They concluded that nearly 50% of their CRPS group had abnormalities of spinothalamic, trigeminothalamic and corticospinal function, which they suggested may represent abnormal function of the medulla. In summary they state:

> The etiology of these abnormalities is unclear but may be associated with prior head and neck trauma or congenital anomalies. Dysfunction in specific areas of the CNS, and we suggest one of these may be the ventral

medulla, may predispose to syndromes of complex regional pain upon peripheral nociceptive input. Specific pathophysiology cannot be determined currently, but mechanisms may involve any number of homeostatic and antinociceptive functions of the brainstem.

Implications of central mechanisms for physiotherapists

An understanding of the maladaptive changes that can occur within the 'scrutinising' CNS is enlightening to both the therapist and the patient. It may, one day, promote an alteration in approach and a broadening of reasoning models as well as open new opportunities for research.

What is becoming increasingly evident is the complexity of the problem and that a search for a single treatable 'nugget' looks increasingly unlikely in conditions like CRPS. Perhaps, for the present time, a more useful stance requires us to:

1. Accept the condition as being highly complex, difficult and perhaps impossible, to provide a single cure for.
2. Be able to see that it is very amenable to skilled multidimensional management approaches (see Brook's chapters and Chapter 8) whose aim is to provide the patient with better coping strategies and improved function and fitness despite the pain. One hope is that considerate therapists will learn how to communicate fully the implications of long term maladaptive nervous system plasticity to the patient and will, themselves, make positive alterations in their prognosis and management as a result. This requires great care and is highly skilled. But...
3. A degree of hope should wisely be maintained. As mentioned already, the considerable potential that the nervous system has to change plastically and adapt in a positive direction, when given the opportunity, may represent the most constructive avenue of therapy and research. Thus...
4. See the patient with established CRPS as containing in large part maladaptive neuroplastic changes that may have the potential to be overridden via good management. This requires a change of strategy from invasive or single modality approaches that attempt to 'fix' a presumed pathology, to those aimed at all the dimensions of the problem, thereby encouraging adaptive restorative changes in the patient's biology, physiology and psychology. It is the opinion here that understanding a cure for complex chronic conditions like CRPS requires a long and intense investigation into natural processes of recovery, healing and change. What is required are new and adaptive plastic changes in response to established maladaptive ones. It would be a major step if biomedicine could shift its attention away from the established, negative, pathology-focused research paradigm to include a more positive one whereby natural recovery physiology is better understood. Once we understand these processes better, we may well start to understand how they can be more efficiently promoted and nurtured.

5. See it as not inevitable, even in those who may be predisposed to it, and therefore preventable with good *early* recognition and good early multidimensional based management whose prime role is to reassure and restore physical confidence as quickly as possible. This requires the early identification of barriers to poor outcome (see Main & Watson Chapter 8, and chapters in Part 1 of Topical Issues in Pain 2). Pain control and pain management are very much a part of early preventive approaches.

> Central pain mechanisms and central information processing mechanisms related to pain remain poorly understood by the general clinical community. Even so, for the first time in the history of medicine, an understanding of central mechanisms involved in pain offers a far better explanation for the frustrating myriad complex and recalcitrant symptoms and symptom behaviours that these patients suffer and have often been blamed for. As the clinical impact of this new knowledge comes to be better understood by the general medical community, patients and their pains are more likely to get a better hearing.

Methods for managing these types of problems are included in this series of volumes and others (for example, see: Wittink & Hoskins-Michel 1997, Harding 1998, Main & Spanswick 2000).

CRPS mechanisms relating to the 'output' systems of the CNS

The greatest focus in the study of the conditions that now fall into the CRPS classification has been the proposed idea that the sympathetic nervous system (SNS) is somehow functioning in an overactive manner. This widely held belief is now thought to be inaccurate (Dotson 1993, Ochoa et al 1993). Incredibly perhaps, it is now mooted by some that sympathetic efferent activity is, if anything, *decreased,* in so called sympathetically related pain states (Devor & Seltzer 1999, Wasner et al 1999)! As far as pain is concerned, the general consensus seems to be that the sympathetic system is not abnormal and is not discharging in an abnormal way. Any variation of sympathetic output that does occur in these patients is, as in anyone, down to the degree of ongoing physical and mental challenges of everyday life. One point to consider though is that the mechanistic scenario that starts a disorder may well be different from the situation that occurs when it is established and investigated. As argued in the previous chapter, there are instances when changes in sympathetic activity may have a role to play in the development of the syndrome.

It was outlined in the 'sampling' section above, that injured sensory fibres, or intact sensory fibres in nerves that have suffered partial nerve injuries, appear to increase their expression of adrenoreceptors in response to injury. Under these circumstances normal rates of sympathetic firing and subsequent

91

release of noradrenaline will cause excitation of afferents leading to pain. Here, the sympathetic nervous system is said to be 'coupled' to the sensory system. If one thinks in a unidimensional way (i.e. not considering other influencing factors), the more noradrenaline released, as in periods of physical or mental stress, the worse the symptoms should become—and the better they should become in periods of calm or low sympathetic activity.

These points deserve reiteration—release of *normal* physiological levels of noradrenaline (and also circulating adrenaline) will result in the initiation of nociceptive activity and hence possible symptoms, if a coupling mechanism is present. In this way it seems rather unfair for the sympathetic system to receive all the attention when, to the best of our knowledge, its behaviour and physiology are quite normal. To remove parts of it surgically, or to immobilise its activities chemically using sympathetic blocking agents, seems to condemn the innocent party unjustly.

This finding that noradrenaline will activate nociceptors that are noradrenaline sensitive and hence cause pain is the current pathophysiological basis thought responsible for the clinical phenomenon described as 'sympathetically maintained pain' (SMP) first proposed by Roberts (1986). He highlighted the requirement of a 'positive' response to a sympathetic block for the diagnosis of SMP. Also, out of this definition, the concept of sympathetically independent pain (SIP) for pain that often has all the hallmarks of being related to a typical 'sympathetic' syndrome but which fails to respond to blocks, evolved (see previous chapter.) Some of the weaknesses and problems associated with this method of diagnosis are discussed in the following chapter.

A major point here, whether the sympathetic nervous system is normal or not, is that there is a mechanism by which it can exacerbate pain in the periphery. This then is an 'output' mechanism of pain generation which has repercussions for therapists. In the first volume of this series, Gifford (1998c p. 84) urged clinicians to consider how their interactions, physical examinations, treatments and physical manipulations and exercises might impact the activity of the sympathetic system. Anything that represents a threat to homeostasis, or is perceived in any way as threatening, will stimulate a sympathetic response and therefore have the potential to aggravate symptoms. Although somewhat unidimensional and 'peripheral,' this model may provide one feasible explanation as to why therapy-related flare-up can occur. It should also make us more aware of important components of the therapeutic alliance (see Noon chapter in Volume 4 of this series), e.g. in providing a model of the problem for the patient that actively tries to decrease any perceived threat and puts the patient at ease.

Micro milieu of the tissues

So far, the focus of the discussion for peripheral mechanisms of pain in CRPS has emphasised the up-regulation of adrenosensitivity following some form of nerve injury. These models of explanation for CRPS and SMP are therefore more relevant to CRPS Type II (causalgia) because the diagnosis requires the presence of a nerve injury. Since CRPS Type I relates to tissue injury, models based on nerve injury are not relevant to its pathogenesis.

Here, but see also the previous chapter's discussions relating to vascular changes, three research findings are discussed that may apply to peripheral input/output mechanisms relevant to CRPS Type I.

First, as mentioned earlier, there is some evidence that sensory nerve endings in inflamed skin may can become sensitised (i.e. cause hyperalgesia) and can discharge (i.e. cause pain) in response to the presence of noradrenaline (see Levine et al 1986, Hu & Zhu 1989, Sato et al 1993). The findings that support this are:

1. If noradrenaline is introduced into inflamed skin in anyone, it increases the level of hyperalgesia and can cause pain.
2. Adrenoreceptor blockers can decrease hyperalgesia.
3. Sympathectomy can partially prevent hyperalgesia occurring (but see below).
4. C fibre nociceptors with receptive fields in inflamed skin acquire an excitatory response to stimulation of the sympathetic chain or to close arterial noradrenaline injections.
5. In the absence of inflammation however, sympathetic outflow does not excite C fibre nociceptors; in fact, it may even suppress their response to brief noxious stimuli.
6. It seems likely from the above that nociceptor end terminals in the inflamed skin express adrenoreceptors, though direct proof is still missing (Michaelis 2000).

Secondly, it has been found that the process of nociceptor sensitisation following injury seems, in part, to require just the physical presence of sympathetic postganglionic terminals (Levine & Reichling 1999). This mechanism can be viewed as essentially 'passive' since there appears to be no need for impulses arriving from sympathetic pathways in the CNS. It is as if the sympathetic terminals act as a physical 'docking station' for some inflammatory chemical agents and that once they have docked in their specific 'receptors' on the terminal a chemical reaction follows that then produces and releases a secondary end product. Chemical agents known to rely on this 'docking' to produce their sensitising effects during inflammation include bradykinin, noradrenaline and nerve growth factor (NGF) (Levine & Reichling 1999). It is known that both bradykinin and noradrenaline interact in this way to produce prostaglandins.

The action of noradrenaline on the very structure that releases it may seem odd. Be aware though that many chemical agents appear to have this 'autocrine' or self-stimulation effect; that is, they act on the very structure from which they were created and released. Thus, impulses arrive down the sympathetic postganglionic neurone cause the release of noradrenaline, which may then dock onto adrenoreceptors on the terminal membrane and cause a further chain of events leading to the release of another chemical agent, in this case prostaglandin I_2!

Thirdly, Gibbins (1992) has added to this discussion with the finding that about 20% of the sympathetic postganglionic fibres to peripheral blood vessels contain substance P which is discharged in response to tissue damage. It is widely accepted that peripherally released substance P is a potent pro-inflammatory mediator. Gibbins (1992) also demonstrated that substance P can cause a slow autocrine depolarisation of postganglionic sympathetic neurons with a possible subsequent release of the prostaglandin PGE2 (McMahon 1991). PGE2 is a well known pro-inflammatory compound.

The above findings support the notion that chemicals 'dumped' by the SNS into peripheral tissues may directly (noradrenaline to nociceptor coupling), or indirectly (stimulates inflammation formation) lead to an increased discharge of sensitised afferents and hence produce pain.

Other evidence to support this includes the finding that, during inflammation, plasma extravasation is reduced post sympathetomy (Janig 1992) and that there is a flow-independent increase in vascular permeability for macromolecules in RSD patients (van Oyen et al 1993)—a feature that indicates ongoing inflammation (see discussion in Chapter 2).

Although these arguments seem convincing, a few workers have demonstrated that the SNS may have an important role in actually inhibiting inflammation—a quite reasonable mechanism if one considers the importance of bringing healing to a halt in order to conserve energy during times of threat/stress. As an example here, Ochoa et al (1993) reported a *reduction* in the flare response following microstimulation of postganglionic efferents in an animal model.

There is modest evidence to suggest that the target tissues alter their responsiveness to sympathetic outflow following tissue damage. These changes may well be normal physiological responses to tissue injury and inflammation, and hence essential parts of the tissue repair processes. Bennett (1999) advises that pathology, i.e. CRPS Type I (SMP), be viewed as a result of normal physiological processes persisting abnormally after healing—hence persistent inflammation and persistent C fibre nociceptor noradrenaline sensitivity. Not only this, but to fit with the occasionally dramatic and massive early manifestation of CRPS Type I, it may also be sometimes worth thinking in terms of maladaptive or 'excessive' physiological responses from the very start.

The complex dynamics of the interaction between the sympathetic nervous system and inflammation and injury, the sensory system, the vascular system, the immune system and perhaps other systems involved in the control of local tissue responses is emerging, but still remains complex, contentious, occasionally contradictory and sometimes unclear.

Sympathetic sprouting

A recent area of interest for the understanding of mechanisms more relevant to CRPS Type II has been the demonstration of sprouting of sympathetic efferents into the dorsal root ganglia following experimental neuronal injury in animal models (see Fig. 3.3a and b). These sympathetic 'sprouts' have been shown to form 'baskets' of nerve filaments that grow round and embrace dorsal root ganglion cell bodies (i.e. cell bodies of sensory cells) whose axons have been experimentally injured distally. The baskets are not present in normal 'non nerve injured' animals and appear to be triggered by the nerve injury. Several neurotrophins have been linked to this process including nerve growth factor (NGF), brain derived neurotrophic factor (BDNF) as well as a family of cytokines (GP–130, IL–6, and leukemia inhibitory factor (LIF), see Ramer et al 1999 for a detailed review.) What the research is starting to show is that this rather strange phenomenon may represent a physical and physicochemical site where the sympathetic nervous system can yet again 'couple' with the sensory system and hence cause symptoms via its activity. According to the review by Ramer et al (1999) the evidence supporting this is quite compelling even though there is still a long way to go. Janig (1999) however has suggested that to be functional these sprouts need to be capable of discharging at 10–15hz and his studies indicate that the sprouts are incapable of such discharge frequencies. Indeed, in an excellent recent review of the role of the sympathetic nervous system in neuropathic pain, Janig and Baron (2001) caution that there are only a very few studies which show that normal physiological activity of sympathetic nerves or normal physiological concentrations of noradrenaline, in animal models, can elicit impulses and hence pain in damaged primary afferent nerve fibres (see next chapter). It seems that most researchers pour on vast quantities of noradrenaline or hyperstimulate the SNS in order to test whether adrenosensitivity occurs! Having said that it has still been shown that normal nerves do not respond to the same large quantities/activities or concentrations.

Finally, from a clinical perspective this dorsal root ganglion 'coupling' site draws attention to a proximal pathophysiological location of a potential pain mechanism. It also further emphasises the difficulties of targeted mechanism based treatment.

Immune based disease?

There has been an increase in the amount of attention that the immune system has received in the pathogenesis of this condition (Thompson 2001, Calder et al 1998, van Oyen et al 1993, Weihe & Nohr 1992). Several cytokines are known to be involved in communication between the immune and nervous systems and include tumor necrosis factor alpha (TNFα), interleukin-6 (IL-6), and leukemia inhibitory factor (LIF). There is little doubt that nervous tissue is not only sensitive to these chemicals but also uses them to determine its responses to injury. They may even be significant factors in governing whether the response is adaptive or maladaptive.

The nervous system is thought to be able to recruit the immune system by influencing specific cell types. The main cell that has been studied here is the macrophage. Macrophages form an important interface between the inflammatory response to injury and the recruitment of the immune system.

95

Intact Preparation

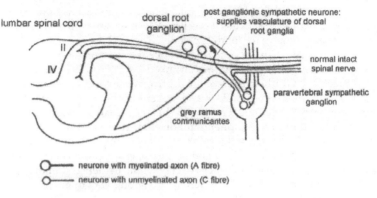

Fig. 3.3a Relation between afferent neurones and their projections in the lumbar outflow. Here, there is no interaction between the sympathetic post ganglionic fibres and the afferent fibres (A and C fibres).

Adapted from: Janig W, McLachlan EM 1994 The role of modifications in noradrenergic peripheral pathways after nerve lesions in the generation of pain. In: Fields HL, Libeskind JC (eds) Pharmacological Approaches to the Treatment of Chronic Pain: new concepts and critical issues. Progress in Pain Research and Management Vol. 1. IASP Press, Seattle

After a peripheral nerve lesion

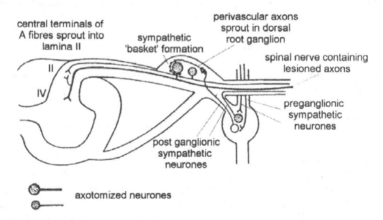

Fig. 3.3b After ligating and cutting the sciatic nerve postganglionic perivascular axons in the dorsal root ganglion area sprout to form basketlike structures around injured neurons cell bodies.

Adapted from: Janig W, McLachlan EM 1994 The role of modifications in noradrenergic peripheral pathways after nerve lesions in the generation of pain. In: Fields HL, Libeskind JC (eds) Pharmacological Approaches to the Treatment of Chronic Pain: new concepts and critical issues. Progress in Pain Research and Management Vol. 1. IASP Press, Seattle

For example, they are known to play an active role in the generation of pain following neuronal damage (Ramar et al 1999, Weihe & Nohr 1992) and they have been shown to have membrane receptors to several neurotransmitters (Weihe & Nohr 1992). This indicates that their activity may be modified in some part by the nervous system. These workers further postulate that other immune cells may have similar receptors.

Weihe and Nohr (1992) have suggested that there may be an interaction between individual neurons (both sensory and sympathetic) and macrophages, lymphocytes and mast cells that reside within the nerve i.e. intrafasicularly. This is an interesting observation as this type of interaction would be impossible to diagnose. These authors also comment that if such a process became established, it may 'spread' more proximally and could involve both the dorsal root ganglion and dorsal horn. They support this hypothesis with findings from biopsied sympathetic ganglia.

Calder et al (1998) have suggested that the sensory-immune interaction may occur in the target tissue. They took skin biopsies from symptomatic areas of patients diagnosed with CRPS Type I (RSD). They used a barrage of immunostaining tests in order to ascertain which cell types were present in the skin. An important point was that there was no macroscopic evidence of inflammation in the areas studied. However, they did find an abundance of Langerhan cells (cells known to be derived from mature macrophages) in their samples. Significantly, these cells are not present in normal skin or in that from patients with other types of neuropathic pain states (McAllistar et al 1996).

Langerhan cells are capable of producing several different types of cytokines including $TNF\alpha$, IL-6 and also the neurotrophin nerve growth factor (NGF). All these compounds are capable of producing pain and changes within sensory neurons (Michaelis 2000).

Calder et al (1998) also suggest that these and related molecules may gain access to the central nervous system and cross the blood-brain barrier producing a more systemic effect and illness behaviours (see Watkins et al 1995 for an in-depth and fascinating account of these processes.)

Recent evidence supports the hypothesis that this condition is in part a neuro-immune disease and, quite likely, a psycho-neuro-immune one, too. This is a fascinating prospect that would go some way to explaining why a mulitifaceted approach to its' management appears to be successful. There is obviously much more work to be performed, but once again we are made aware of the need for paradigms that are inclusive of such concepts!

Conclusion

This chapter and the last have reviewed some of the significant recent research findings into the mechanisms thought responsible for CRPS. This chapter has placed the overview of mechanisms within the context of the 'sampling–scrutinising–responding' circle proposed in the Mature Organism Model (Gifford 1998), and as a result has considered potential points of interest at the sensory nerve terminals, along the sensory nerve, within the central nervous system at all levels and finally focuses on the impact that some of the output systems may play.

- The idea that CRPS relates purely to sympathetic dysfunction or abnormality is challenged powerfully. Clinicians are urged to be cautious and to consider the problem as not having a specific pathological site to target.
- The notion that there is a useful medical cure for the problem has to be considered very carefully (see next two chapters). There are probably only a few real clinical experts in the world who have a good broad understanding of all the issues and are highly skilled at blocking procedures. As the reader will find out in the next chapter, many of the procedures that medicine has to offer are dramatic, invasive, not necessarily guaranteed, and based on unproven unidimensional models that usually target the SNS, which in all probability is quite normal. Referring patients on to inappropriate and possibly inexperienced specialists, and thus over-medicalising the disorder, needs to be considered very carefully with the present state of knowledge (see Chapter 4).
- The problem is more than just pain, swelling and stiffness; it invariably involves a very physically disabled and unhappy patient. Considering the multidimensional impact of the problem and all facets of it in relation to the patient's life should guide better management strategies.

ENDNOTE

[1] Second order cells in the dorsal horn have many names and may be a source of confusion. They are also known as: transmission, or 'T' cells; wide dynamic range cells (WDR); nociceptive specific cells (NS); or simply, dorsal horn cells. Their cell bodies lie in the dorsal horn and their axons may then communicate with other nerve cells at many levels. This may be locally, segmentally, intersegmentally, or beyond up to the brain where further synapsing, scrutinising and processing occurs.

REFERENCES

Bennett GJ, Roberts WJ 1996 Animal models and their contribution to our understanding of complex regional pain syndrome I and II. In: Janig W, Stanton-Hicks M (eds) Reflex Sympathetic Dystrophy: A Reappraisal. IASP Press, Seattle

Bennett GJ 1999 Scientific basis for the evaluation and treatment of RSD/CRPS syndromes: Laboratory studies in animals and man. In: Max M (ed) Pain 1999—an updated review. Refresher course syllabus. IASP Press, Seattle 331–337

Blumberg H 1992 Clinical and pathophysiological aspects of reflex sympathetic dystrophy and sympathetic maintained pain pathway. In: Janig W, Schmidt R F (eds) Reflex Sympathetic Dystrophy. Pathophysiological Mechanisms and Clinical Implications. VCH, Weinheim

Calder JS, Holten I, McAllister RMR 1998 Evidence for immune system involvement in reflex sympathetic dystrophy. Journal of Hand Surgery 23B (2):147–150

Campbell JN, Meyer RA, Raja SN 1992 Is nociceptor activation by alpha-1 adrenoreceptors the culprit in sympathetically maintained pain? American Pain Society Journal 1:3–11

Coderre TJ, Basbaum AI, Levine JD 1989 Neural control of vascular permeability: interactions between primary afferents, mast cells, and sympathetic efferents. Journal of Neurophysiology 62: 48–58

Coderre TJ, Katz J, Vaccarino AI, Melzack R 1993 Contribution of central neuroplasticity to pathological pain: review of clinical and experimental evidence. Pain 52: 259–282

Devor M 1991 Neuropathic pain and injured nerve: peripheral mechanisms In: Wells JCD, Woolf CJ (eds) Pain Mechanisms and Management. British Medical Bulletins 47 (3):619–630

Devor M 1994 The pathophysiology of damaged peripheral nerves. In: Wall PD, Melzack R (eds) Textbook of Pain 3rd edn. Churchill Livingstone, Edinburgh

Devor M 1996 Pain mechanisms and pain syndromes. In: Campbell JN (ed) Pain 1996—an updated review. IASP Press, Seattle

Devor M, Seltzer Z 1999 The pathophysiology of damaged peripheral nerves in relation to chronic pain. In: Wall PD, Melzack R (eds) Textbook of Pain 4th edn. Churchill Livingstone, Edinburgh

Doubell TP, Mannion RJ, Woolf CJ 1999 The dorsal horn: state dependent sensory processing, plasticity and the generation of pain. In: Wall PD, Melzack R (eds) Textbook of Pain 4th edn. Churchill Livingstone, Edinburgh

Doupe J, Cullen CH, Chance GQ 1944 Post traumatic pain and the causalgic syndrome. Journal of Neurology and Psychiatry 7:33–48

Dotson R 1993 Causalgia—reflex sympathetic dystrophy–sympathetically maintained pain: myth and reality. Muscle and Nerve 16:1049–1055

Drummond PD 1995 Noradrenaline increases hyperalgesia to heat in skin sensitized by capsaicin. Pain 60: 311–315

Drummond PD, Finch PM, Gibbins I 1996 Innervation of hyperalgesic skin in patients with complex regional pain syndrome. The Clinical Journal of Pain 12 (3): 222–231

Dubner R, Ruda M A 1992 Activity-dependent neuronal plasticity following tissue injury and inflammation. Trends in Neuroscience 15: 96–103

Eliav E, Herzberg U, Ruda MA, Bennett GJ 1999 Neuropathic pain from an experimental neuritis of the rat sciatic nerve. Pain 83 (2): 169–182

Fields, HL Basbaum, AI 1999 Central nervous system mechanisms of pain modulation. In: Wall PD, Melzack R (eds) Textbook of Pain 4th edn. Churchill Livingstone, Edinburgh 309–329

Galer BS, Bruehl S, Harden RN 1998 IASP diagnostic criteria for complex regional pain. a preliminary empirical validation study. The Clinical Journal of Pain 14:48–54

Gibbins I 1992 The final common sympathetic pathway. In: Janig W, Schmidt RF (eds) Reflex Sympathetic Dystrophy. Pathophysiological Mechanisms and Clinical Implications. VCH, Weinheim

Gifford LS 1998 The mature organism model. In: Gifford LS (ed) Topical Issues in Pain. Whiplash—science and management. Fear-avoidance beliefs and behaviour. CNS Press, Falmouth 45–56

Gifford LS 1998a Tissue and input related mechanisms. In: Gifford LS (ed) Topical Issues in Pain 1. Whiplash—science and management. Fear-avoidance beliefs and behaviour. CNS Press, Falmouth 57–65

Gifford LS 1998b Central mechanisms. In: Gifford LS (ed) Topical Issues in Pain 1. Whiplash—science and management. Fear-avoidance beliefs and behaviour. CNS Press, Falmouth 67–80

Gifford LS 1998c Output mechanisms. In: Gifford LS (ed) Topical Issues in Pain 1. Whiplash—science and management. Fear-avoidance beliefs and behaviour. CNS Press, Falmouth 81–91

Granit R, Skoglund CR 1945 Facilitation, inhibition and depression at the 'artificial synapse' formed by the cut end of a mammalian nerve. Journal of Physiology (Lond) 103: 435–448

Habler HJ, Janig W, Koltzenberg M 1987 Activation of unmyelinated afferents in chronically lesioned nerves by adrenaline and excitation of sympathetic efferents in cats. Neurocience Letters 82:35–40

Harding V 1998 Application of the cognitive-behavioural approach. In: Pitt-Brooke J (ed) Rehabilitation of Movement. WB Saunders, London

Hu S, Zhu J 1989 Sympathetic facilitation of sustained discharges of polymodal nociceptors. Pain 38: 85–90

Janig W 1990 Activation of afferent fibres ending in old neuromas by sympathetic stimulation in the rat. Neuroscience Letters 111: 309–311

Janig W 1992 Can reflex sympathetic dystrophy be reduced to an alpha-adrenoreceptor disease? American Pain Society Journal 1 (1):16–22

Janig W 1993 Pain and the autonomic nervous system: pathophysiological mechanisms. In: Bannister R, Mathias CJ (eds) Autonomic Failure 3rd edn. Oxford University Press, Oxford

Janig W 1996 The puzzle of 'reflex sympathetic dystrophy': mechanisms, hypothesis, open questions. In: Janig W, Stanton-Hicks M (eds) Reflex Sympathetic Dystrophy: A Reappraisal. IASP Press, Seattle

Janig W 1999 Personal communication. IASP conference Vienna

Janig W, Baron R 2001 The role of the sympathetic nervous system in neuropathic pain: Clinical observations and animal models. In: Hansson PT, Fields HL, Hill RG, Marchettini P (eds) Neuropathic Pain: Pathophysiology and Treatment, Progress in Pain Research and Management, Vol 21. IASP Press, Seattle 125–149

Koltzenburg M 1996 Afferent mechanisms mediating pain and hyperalgesias in neuralgia. In: Janig W, Stanton-Hicks M (eds) Reflex Sympathetic Dystrophy: A Reappraisal. IASP Press, Seattle

Levine JD, Taiwo YO, Collins SD, Tam JK 1986 Noradrenaline hyperalgesia. Nature 323: 158–160

Levine JD, Reichling DB 1999 Peripheral mechanisms of inflammatory pain. In: Wall PD, Melzack R (eds) Textbook of Pain 4th edn. Churchill Livingstone, Edinburgh 59–84

Lisney SJW 1992 Pathophysiological properties of afferent fibres after nerve injury and their possible significance to reflex sympathetic dystrophy. In: Janig W, Schmidt RF (eds) Reflex Sympathetic Dystrophy. Pathophysiological Mechanisms and Clinical Implications. VCH, Weinheim

Main CJ, Spanswick CC 2000 Pain Management. An interdisciplinary approach. Churchill Livingstone, Edinburgh

Maves TJ, Pechman PS, Gebhart GF, Meller ST 1993 Possible chemical contributions from chromic gut sutures produces disorders of pain sensation like those seen in man. Pain 54: 57–69

McAllistar RMR, Terenghi G, Calder JS 1996 Reinnervation of the skin following peripheral nerve division in man: a quantitative study. European Journal of Neurology 3 (Suppl 5): 212

McMahon S B 1991 Mechanisms of sympathetic pain. In: Wells JCD, Woolf CJ (eds) Pain Mechanisms and Management. British Medical Bulletins 47 (3):619–630

McMahon SB 1992 Dorsal horn plasticity and reflex sympathetic dystrophy. In: Janig W, Schmidt RF (eds) Reflex Sympathetic Dystrophy. Pathophysiological Mechanisms and Clinical Implications. VCH, Weinheim

McMahon SB, Koltzenburg M 1990 Novel Classes of Nociceptors: Beyond Sherrington. Trends in Neuroscience 13:199–201

McMahon SB, Koltzenburg M 1990a The changing role of primary afferent neurons in pain. Pain 43: 269–272

McMahon SB, Lewin GR, Wall PD 1993 central hyperexcitability triggered by noxious inputs. Current Opinion in Neurobiology 3:602–610

Michaelis M 2000 Coupling of sympathetic and somatosensory neurons following nerve injury: mechanisms and potential significance for the generation of pain. In: Devor M, Rowbotham MC, Wiesenfeld-Hallin (eds) Proceedings of the 9th Congress on Pain Research and Management. IASP Press, Seattle

Ochoa JL, Yarnitsky D, Marchettini P, Dotson R, Cline M 1993 Interactions between sympathetic vasoconstrictor outflow and c nociceptor induced antidromic vasoconstriction. Pain 54:191–196

Petrovic P, Ingvar M 2002 Imaging cognitive modulation of pain processing. Pain 95: 1–5

Ramar M, Thompson SWN, McMahon SB 1999 Causes and consequences of sympathetic basket formation in dorsal root ganglia. Pain (Suppl. 6) S111–S120

Roberts WJ 1986 A hypothesis on the physiological basis for causalgia and related pains. Pain 24:297–311

Rose S 1992 The Making of Memory: From molecules to mind. Bantam Press, London

Sato J, Suzuki S, Iseki T, Kumazawa T 1993 Adrenergic excitation of cutaneous nociceptors in chronically inflamed rats. Neuroscience Letters 164: 225–228

Schwartzman RJ, McLelland TL 1987 Reflex sympathetic dystrophy. Archives of Neurology 44:555–561

Stanton-Hicks M, Janig W, Hassenbusch S, Haddox J D, Boas R, Wilson P 1995 Reflex sympathetic dystrophy: changing concepts and taxonomy. Pain 63:127–133

Thimineur M, Saberski L 1996 Complex regional pain syndrome Type I (RSD) or peripheral mononeuropathy? A discussion of three cases. Clinical Journal of Pain 12:145–150

Thimineur M, Sood P, Kravitz E, Gudin J, Kitaj M 1998 Central nervous system abnormalities in complex regional pain syndrome (CRPS): clinical and quantitative evidence of medullary dysfunction. Clinical Journal of Pain 14: 256–267

Thompson SWN 2001 Is the sympathetic nervous system a pain? Neuroscience News 4 (3):35–41

Van Houdenhove B, Vasquez G, Onghena P, Stans L, Vandeput C, Vermaut G, Vervaeke G, Igodt P, Vertommen H 1992 Etiopathogenesis of reflex sympathetic dystrophy: a review and biopsychosocial hypothesis. Clinical Journal of Pain 8(4):300–306

Van Oyen WJG, Arntz IE, Claessens AMJ, van der Meer JWM, Corstens FHM, Goris RJA 1993 Reflex sympathetic dystrophy of the hand: an excessive inflammatory response? Pain 55: 151–157

Wall PD 1995 Noreadrenaline-evoked pain in neuralgia. Pain 63:1–2

Wall PD, Gutnik M 1974 Ongoing activity in peripheral nerves: the physiology and pharmacology of impulses originating from a neuroma. Experimental Neurology 43:580–593

Wall PD, Gutnik M 1974a Properties of afferent nerve impulse from a neuroma. Nature 248: 740–743

Wasner G, Heckman K, Maier C, Baron R 1999 Vascular abnormalities in acute reflex sympathetic dystrophy (CRPS 1). Archives of Neurology 56:613–620

Watkins LR, Maier SF, Goehler HE 1995 Immune activation and the role of pro-inflammatory cytokines in inflammation, illness responses and pathological pain conditions. Pain 63: 289–302

Weihe E, Nohr D 1992 A neuroimmune sensory-sympathetic link in the pathophysiology and chronic pain cycle of " reflex sympathetic dystrophy" (RSD). In: Janig W, Schmidt RF (eds) Reflex Sympathetic Dystrophy. Pathophysiological Mechanisms and Clinical Implications. VCH, Weinheim.

Wittink H, Hoskins-Michel T 1997 Chronic Pain Management for Physical Therapists. Butterworth Heinemann, Boston

101

Woolf CJ 1992 Maladaptive neuronal plasticity and reflex sympathetic dystrophy. In: Janig W, Schmidt RF (eds) Reflex Sympathetic Dystrophy. Pathophysiological Mechanisms and Clinical Implications. VCH, Weinheim

Woolf CJ 1994 The dorsal horn: state-dependent sensory processing and the generation of pain. In: Wall, PD, Melzack R (eds) Textbook of Pain 3rd edn. Churchill Livingstone, Edinburgh

Woolf CJ, Thompson SWN 1991 The induction and maintenance of central sensitisation is dependent on N-methyl-D-aspartic acid receptor activation: implications for the treatment of post injury pain hypersensitivity states. Pain 44: 293–29

4

Sympathetically maintained pain: myth or reality?

MICK THACKER AND LOUIS GIFFORD

Introduction

Sympathetically maintained pain (SMP) is often assumed to be the major feature of complex regional pain syndrome; it may not be. Also, and perhaps to the detriment of the patient who has the condition, a focus on the sympathetic system seems to underpin the diagnostic and therapeutic decision-making.

SMP is a controversial topic with some authorities now seriously questioning its existence. As already described in Chapters 2 and 3, involvement of the sympathetic nervous system (SNS) in the generation of pain and other symptoms can be suspected from patient's presentation. There is a commonly held belief that changes in blood flow, altered skin colouration and disturbance of sweating are a result of SNS involvement. Hopefully the reviews in the last two chapters indicate that this stance, though reasonable, may need tempering. Thompson (2001) recently wrote 'the direct involvement of the SNS has perhaps been overestimated at the detriment of other indirect mechanisms,' suggesting that we may have focused on what appear obvious explanations at the expense of more involved mechanisms.

Simple explanations have many advantages but we must guard against complacency. Pat Wall (1999) once said: 'It is almost impossible to replace widely accepted medical dogmas, especially where the paradigm being challenged has to be replaced with a more complicated one!'

Paramedical professionals have been accused of over diagnosing CRPS Type I (Janig 1996). This over diagnosis appears to be based on their assumption that they are observing signs of sympathetic dysfunction, which is now thought to be erroneous in the light of current research. Janig (1996) states that 'it is impossible to implicate the sympathetic nervous system in the production of signs and symptoms from physical examination alone.' It is important that we realise the full implication of research for clinical diagnosis and the potentially dangerous repercussions for our patients, such as requests for invasive blocking procedures and continued investigation (see next chapter) when they may be highly inappropriate.

History

Roberts (1986) is widely acknowledged as the originator of the term Sympathetically Maintained Pain. It appears that he was heavily influenced by the seminal work of Livingstone, in particular his viscous circle hypothesis (Livingstone 1943). Briefly, this stated that pain led to alterations in sympathetic discharge leading to a decrease in circulation and to muscle spasm that resulted in further pain.

Together with several co-workers, Roberts performed numerous experiments to investigate the role of the sympathetic nervous system (SNS) in the generation of pain. His findings led him to describe a mechanism by which painful input to the nervous system is maintained (and generated) by activities of the SNS.

Over a decade before Robert's work, Wall and Gutnik (1974, 1974a) demonstrated that damaged sensory nerve fibres showed an increased sensitivity to adrenaline and noradrenaline. Around the same time John Hannington-Kiff (1974) had described the successful use of guanethidine, a drug known to inhibit noradrenaline release from sympathetic neurones, to relieve the pain of patients suffering from reflex sympathetic dystrophy. It is interesting to note that none of these authorities deemed it fit to suggest that their findings revealed a novel pain mechanism.

Since Robert's (1986) work there has been an enormous amount of 'space' devoted to the controversy of whether there is such a phenomenon as SMP. More recently there have been increasing attempts to clarify the clinical situation. Such attempts have faced many confounding findings, including the observation that sympathectomy can actually lead to *increased* pain and associated epiphenomena that are usually ascribed to sympathetic over-activity (Perl 1994, Kramis et al 1996).

At present there is a widely held belief that SMP represents a condition of altered sensitivity to noradrenaline (Campbell et al 1992, 1994) with central repercussions. The underlying peripheral mechanism is thought to be due to upregulation of adrenoreceptors in peripheral nervous tissue (Campbell et al 1992, 1994; see also previous chapter). The result of this is a peripheral increase in sensitivity to noradrenaline whose presence then drives an increased afferent barrage into the CNS. Changes in central sensitivity follow the afferent barrage. The vicious circle hypothesis then predicts that the central sensitisation leads to an increased sympathetic output, thus promoting the release of noradrenaline, and thereby completing the out–to in–to out positive feedback 'circle.'

This chapter attempts to offer a balanced account of the topic and to highlight the clinical points for the practising therapist. The majority of the chapter focuses on human studies as these are thought most relevant for the clinician, but some animal work is included in order to give a full picture of current thinking.

Sympathetic blocks

For most clinicians SMP may only be suspected from the clinical history since it cannot be identified via features of pain, history, or standard physical testing. Currently, the only known way of identifying it is to perform a 'sympathetic block' and see if the patient's pain, or a component of the patient's pain, is quickly relieved (Campbell et al 1992, 1994). Recall from Chapter 2 that pain can be viewed as being 'sympathetically independent' (SIP) and that a given patient may have varying proportions of SIP and SMP.

The introduction of the sympathetic blocking agent guanethidine into the clinical management of CRPS Type I (RSD) by Hannington-Kiff (1974) was mentioned above. Guanethidine has its actions by causing the postganglionic sympathetic neurons to discharge their stores of noradrenaline and ultimately to reduce its concentrations within the nerve so that it becomes impotent to later stimulation. (*Clinical Note: In those with adrenosensitivity if the guanethidine block is performed without local anaesthetic, the initial 'discharge' of noradrenaline can lead to marked increases in pain until the noradrenaline is washed away by the circulation.*) Not only does guanethidine 'empty' the stores of noradrenaline, it also delays any re-uptake of the released chemical by the sympathetic nerve fibres.

Recently the efficacy of guanethidine and related compounds as therapeutic agents (reviewed in Glynn et al 1993, McQuay & Moore 1998, and Kingery 1997), and as diagnostic tools has been challenged. For example, in his extensive review of treatment trials for CRPS, Kingery (1997) states that '...intravenous regional blocks with guanethidine are ineffective analgesics compared to placebo or no treatment.' One of the trials cited in the review is described here:

Ramamurthy and Hoffman (1995) randomised 60 CRPS patients to receive either up to four regional guanethidine blocks with lignocaine (local anaesthetic), or to a patient control group that received an injection of lignocaine and saline only. The results revealed that there was no difference in outcome between the guanethidine and the control groups. Also, patients in all groups showed a decrease in oedema, as well as sweating, trophic and vasomotor changes. All those in the guanethidine group had at least one block and those receiving up to four blocks had no greater degree of pain relief.

These findings strikingly show that the effectiveness of guanethidine blocks for presumed SMP, as well as non-pain related clinical features that may be associated with sympathetic impairment, can be manipulated just as effectively with a local anaesthetic whose normally short lived effects most of us have witnessed after dental care! It also adds credibility to the idea that the patient's own system may have the ways and means of achieving positive change given the right inputs or triggers. These may be injections but could also be any variety of non-invasive treatments too.

Supporters of sympathetic blocking procedures may counter findings like these by stating that multiple blocks are sometimes needed to produce a good outcome and that the trials only offer one, or a few at best. It is staggering to find that there are various reports suggesting that anywhere from 1 to over 300 blocks may be required for successful therapeutic effect (Wynn-Parry 1996). The main issue is surely that proponents of multiple blocks need to come up with better evidence harvested from much higher quality trials than are currently available.

The results of reviews of trials like those cited above challenge clinicians to think very carefully before referring patients for guanethidine blocks or any blocking procedures. Physiotherapists are often asked by patients for their opinion regarding such procedures. The advice here is that we should provide honest answers that are based on the results and findings of well structured double blind trials like those above.

However, although challenged (see Kingery 1997), many other sympathetic blocking agents that are reported do have some validity in the management of presumed SMP. For example Baron et al (1999a) reported that 85% of patients showed positive early responses to blocking procedures, but that this figure reduced to 42% at follow up 1–6 months later.

Whether the success of blocking procedures is sufficient to establish the existence of SMP has to be seen in the light of interesting alternative explanations for their effect:

- Phentolamine is an alpha adrenoreceptor antagonist. Its supporters suggest that its use is superior to that of other blocking agents and recommend its use for the determination of the presence of SMP (Campbell et al 1992, 1994). However, the emerging picture regarding phentolamine's specific blocking action at the adrenoreceptor is slightly less clear than originally conceived. There is now evidence that it may be responsible for relief of pain via its sodium ion channel blocking action. Sodium ion channels have a well established role in the propagation of impulses and in the production of pain (Dotson 1993, Bennett 1999, Black et al 2001). This means that phentolamine should be effective for a great many more classes and mechanisms of pain.
- Other components that could account for the effectiveness of blocking agents include its method of delivery. For example, there are data to suggest that both saline and the application of a tourniquet can have similar short term outcomes to the infiltration of an active compound (Janig 1992, Kingery 1997, Price at al 1996, Bennett 1999). Either or both of these technical aspects could account for early, post block, pain relief and hence result in a false positive result for SMP. For those who may be puzzled by this, it is important to consider on the one hand the placebo effect (see below and Volume 4 in this series), and on the other that

compression or squeezing, as in the tourniquet test, is a common way of relieving pain in all of us. It probably has its effect via classic, simple peripherally induced (increased Aβ fibre activity) gate control.

- Price and co-workers (Price et al 1996, 1998) have focused on the difficulties of separating 'true' responses from those of placebo in the identification of SMP. They published an excellent paper comparing the effects of local anaesthetic blocks with saline in CRPS Type I patients (Price et al 1998). They were able to show that both interventions relieved pain, but the duration of pain relief was longer with the local anaesthetic.

In their 1998 paper, Price and colleagues raise several important points that illustrate how difficult it is to pinpoint a pain mechanism based on a comparison of results of any intervention. First, they noted that both saline and the sympathetic blocking anaesthetic relieved pain. Since saline does not block the sympathetic system this demonstrates that saline relieves the pain via a different process. It also suggests that the pain may not be sympathetically maintained at all. However the sympathetic blocks do change sweating and skin temperature, which are measures of sympathetic activity, whereas the saline showed no effect on this.

An important message from this is that alterations to signs and symptoms following diagnostic procedures, or any treatments that are assumed to be targeting the SNS, *do not necessarily* indicate that they really are! Unfortunately we simply cannot make totally confident judgements about a given source or mechanism of pain or any other symptom, based on the outcome of interventions and treatments. This applies to biomedical interventions just as much as to physiotherapy techniques and treatments applied to any condition. The idea that a 'localised' technique has only a local effect needs revision. Modulation of pain via modulation of nervous system activity is a complex process that is unlikely to be resolved to a single process even though it may appear so. It seems that altering the input to the system, from virtually anywhere, by virtually anything, may be capable of modulating the output! It is important to reason that all interventions have a multidimensional impact. For example, in the physiotherapy process the integration of things like exercises, examinations, advice, manipulations, skill acquisitions and even demonstrations may all consciously or subconsciously change an individual's perception or relevance of a particular feature of a condition and this may be enough to alter the expression of the system. It is possible that many of the benefits of a multidimensional reasoning model and approach in physiotherapy, for SMP or virtually any other pain condition, has its role by affecting all components of the patient's pain. This may be why attempts to isolate treatment effects in well controlled research trials fail to demonstrate clear benefits. The very structure and nature of a clinical trial seems to result in the intervention being unnaturally severed from the sum total of the therapeutic interaction (see the Noon 2002 chapter in Volume 4 of this series) and the benefits of the 'psychosocial placebo' described in by Richard Shortall in the same volume (Shortall 2002).

This section has discussed some of the challenges that surround the assumptions about diagnostic and therapeutic blocking. Clearly, the foundations of the procedures are not proving to be as substantial as they once were thought to be. Sympathetic involvement in pain generation is still taken seriously however and the challenge for medical research may be to find more water-tight diagnostic testing procedures and, by understanding pain mechanism and pain processing better, to devise more potent treatment protocols. The news is not all bad for drug management. For example, the successful trials of the use of systemic drugs such as clonidine and prazocin (alpha adrenoreceptor antagonists) in the management of CRPS Type I patients still supports the concept of sympathetic involvement and this pharmacological route for pain management (Schwartzman & McClellan 1987). A simple plea would be for those who advocate a pharmacological management paradigm to start to appreciate that other dimensions of pain and physical function relevant to the patient's life need attention at the same time.

A note on sympathectomies

As far back as 1916 Leriche (cited in Scadding 1999) described the relief of pain, sweating changes and skin discoloration following sympathectomy of patients with causalgia. Apparently, the causalgia in the first patient he described was caused by a brachial plexus injury and thrombosis of the brachial artery. The sympathectomy performed involved resecting the adventitia of a length of the brachial artery. Later, this 'peri-arterial sympathectomy' was replaced by preganglionic sympathectomy for the treatment of painful nerve injuries sustained by soldiers during the two World Wars. The relief of causalgic pain by sympathectomy lead to the assumption that the sympathetic system was involved in its pathogenesis. But, there was no critical evaluation of its effectiveness. Since this time, sympathectomy has been a common treatment for causalgia and RSD. A commonly repeated statement regarding efficacy of sympathectomy runs '...it is recognised by those regularly treating these patients that while temporary pain relief may occur, long-term results are poor...leading most to abandon the procedures' (see Scadding 1999). That pain frequently returned after sympathectomy led to the assumption that the original sympathectomy had been incomplete or that a new sympathetic innervation had occurred. Animal experiments suggest another cause: that sympathectomy itself may induce SMP (Bennett & Roberts 1996)! These animal studies show that injury to sympathetic postganglionic fibres may induce a situation where intact C fibre nociceptors become adrenosensitive and that sympathectomy may induce the same phenomenon. Bennett and Roberts (1996) suggest that returned pain or increased pain and often new proximal pain that follows after sympathectomy be described as a new syndrome: 'postsympathectomy neuralgia'!

While sympathectomy is not a good treatment option, the results of sympathectomy do suggest that the SNS is involved in production and maintenance of pain.

Rekindling of pain via sympathetic agents or sympathetic stimulation

Further support for the existence of SMP comes from the well cited observation that following successful sympathetic blocking (pain relief), the designated SMP can be rekindled by the introduction of an 'alpha adrenoreceptor agonist' (e.g. noradrenaline) into the area of pain relief. The noradrenaline 'agonist' is introduced either by injecting under the skin or iontophoretically (Torebjork et al 1995, Ali 2000).

The reasoning here is that if pain is maintained sympathetically, it should be relieved by blocking the sympathetic system, but also should be re-established with the return of the stimulating agent produced by the sympathetic system. It is interesting to note that only 28% (seven of 25) of the SMP diagnosed patients in the Torebjork et al (1995) study (diagnosed by a positive response to sympathetic block) responded with an *increase* in pain following injection of noradrenaline into an area of sensitive skin. This is quite a discrepancy. However, in their study they noted that noradrenaline applied to the skin in all 10 patients with sympathetically *independent* pain (SIP), had no effect on the pain. Clearly, the relative proportion of patients responding to a noradrenaline challenge was higher in the SMP group than the SIP group. A greater number of patient trials may help clarify the situation.

Why is it though, that in some patients with SMP the pain can be made worse or brought back by the introduction of noradrenaline (the seven), while in others (the remaining 18) it cannot? As ever, thoughtful and considered (potential) explanations for this finding were offered by Wall (1995). He suggested that these patients might have already had all their available adrenoreceptors 'occupied' preventing further pain exacerbation when noradrenaline was introduced. Simply, the noradrenaline had no available receptor targets to act on. Alternatively the actual adrenosensitive structures could be sited deeper than the skin and therefore would be unlikely to respond to the subdermal injection or the iontophoresis. Another possibility suggested was that these individuals may have had a different focus of their adrenosensitivity; perhaps the portion of their nervous system sensitive to adrenaline was more centrally placed - on the dorsal root ganglion cell bodies of the affected fibres (see Chapter 3). Wall (1995) pointed out that there may be a subset of patients who, as a result of having this more proximally situated site of adrenosensitivity, might be incorrectly diagnosed as having SIP following a negative response to guanethidine blocking. Recall that guanethidine block only immobilises the SNS in the limb where it is introduced. Thus, patients with only a proximal 'dorsal root ganglion' site

109

of noradrenaline sensitivity, may be wrongly diagnosed as 'SIP' following a negative response to guanethidine block. However, a sympathetic block applied to the ganglion on the sympathetic chain *would* immobilise the SNS supply to the dorsal root ganglion which would then produce the relief and hence the SMP diagnosis. Thus, negative responses to a *peripheral* blocks are not 100% reliable in indicating that SMP is *not* present.

In their patient study, Torebjork et al (1995) found that all but one of the 12 patients they followed up, converted from having SMP in the early stages, to having SIP at reassessment many years later. Also, most of those who were made worse by noradrenaline in the early stages, when they were 'SMP,' were shown to be unaffected by it at the later time, when they were 'SIP.'

Again Wall (1995) offers a commentary suggesting that damaged sensory nerves may well undergo 'phenotypic' switches. In other words, they change their structural make-up over time and as a result change their sensitivity states. For example, initially their cell walls may be well endowed with a high population of active adrenoreceptors, but later on the numbers drop away significantly. As Wall (1995) puts it, there is a '...plasticity in which they [the damaged nerves] evolve from one pathological state to another.' Things change and move as time goes on. Wall (1995) reports that in animal studies of experimentally produced peripheral nerve injury he and Devor '...observe a striking period of adrenaline sensitivity which lasts only from the period 1 week after the lesion to 3 weeks after the lesion.' He introduces the idea of 'temporary adrenaline sensitivity'. He also pleads for longer term studies to be done and notes that in those animal studies of nerve injury that have looked longer, they all resolve spontaneously unlike the majority of human cases which do not.

Does this mean that given the right conditions early on, human nerve injury could resolve too? What might these conditions be? Could the biological impact of psychosocial factors that so powerfully predict poor outcome play a part in setting up or facilitating unnecessary long term changes? For example, fear of pain, focus on pain, and the consequent immobility that sometimes occurs may promote plastic changes that favour the pain mechanisms rather than pain inhibition and dampening. Or is there such a difference in make up between rats and humans that we may have to learn to live with the sometimes devastating consequences of long term nerve injury?

For clinicians who administer blocking agents, the finding that pain mechanisms can change and shift with time indicates that they are in a limited position to be able to indicate confidently not only who will benefit, but also, when the benefit will occur.

If one can trust the validity of findings from dated literature it is interesting to note that Walker and Nulson (1948) showed that electrical stimulation of the sympathetic chain led to an increase in pain in those suffering SMP, with no effect on those demonstrating SIP. These findings were reproduced some years later by White and Sweet (1969).

An elegant study performed jointly in Germany and America by Baron and co-workers (Baron et al 1999) assessed the effect of sympathetic stimulation on pain induced by sensitisation of primary afferent C fibres in humans. They produced experimental pain by the infiltration of capsaicin (the chemical responsible for producing the heat sensation from chili peppers) into the skin. This is known to produce a typical pain presentation including spontaneous pain, hyperalgesia, and an axon reflex induced vasodilation. They recorded the individuals' pain reports (intensity), axon reflex (via laser doppler flowometry), size of flare, and area of hyperalgesia. The skin temperature at the recording site was kept constant but they used a thermal 'body-suit' to allow them to produce whole body cooling or warming in order to alter sympathetic discharge.

Their results demonstrated no differences in any of the scores between high and low sympathetic discharge states. This suggests that the sympathetic system is not capable of altering the pain response in this experimental paradigm. The authors are correctly reluctant to over state the importance of their findings in the debate over the existence of SMP. They point out that their study was performed on normal subjects and freely recognise that the changes seen in clinical conditions are different.

Their results would appear to be in contrast to those published earlier by Drummond (1995). He demonstrated that sympathetic discharge increased the reporting of hyperalgesia (following the application of capsaicin) and concluded that sympathetic activity increases pain from the skin. The contrast in results may be due to the differences in the experimental paradigms used. It is interesting to note that Baron et al (1999) did not cite the Drummond (1995) paper.

This example is included for several reasons. First, in depth reviews of this topic consistently produce differing results. Secondly, the results of studies are often affected by even small differences in experimental design; and lastly, literature reviews often fail to identify previous work even when of high relevance. The reader is therefore urged to attempt to maintain a healthy circumspection and scepticism when reading any account even when it has undergone peer review and is written by experts—and that includes these authors!

To end this subsection, it is worth noting that in their editorial, Max and Gilron (1999) suggest that much of the work discussed above should, at least, modify the concept of SMP and the basis of current management. For example, they recommend that the results of Baron et al (1999) call into question the practice of permanent ablation of the sympathetic nervous system until a better methodology is in place to determine who exactly, if anyone, is likely to benefit from such procedures.

Animal studies

Conclusions from animal studies are complicated and unfortunately do not provide a definitive answer or easily stated case either way to the question raised in this chapter. However, the weight of the research findings and the inferences of internationally recognised experts in the field seems to favour the existence of SMP in animal models.

Nerve lesion models

Most of the animal studies into SMP involve surgically produced nerve lesions followed by interventions that impact the sympathetic supply. Interventions that target the SNS include surgical or chemical sympathectomy or the application of adrenoreceptor blocking agents or adrenoreceptor agonists. Changes in pain behaviour and changes in sensitivity to mechanical forces or temperature are then tested/observed. A common protocol is to perform some kind of sympathetic blocking procedure, and then, if the pain behaviour and hyperalgesia is diminished or relieved, to see if it can be rekindled by later introducing noradrenaline, or by chemically, physically, or electrically stimulating the sympathetic system.

Since the models used involve nerve lesions their findings are relevant to CRPS Type II only. Work on animal models relating to CRPS Type I is discussed later.

There are several types of experimental lesion models (see Baron et al 1999, Cepeda 1995, Bennett and Roberts 1996, Bennett 1999).

1. *Ligation and transection.* Here, a peripheral nerve, usually either the sciatic or the saphenous nerves, is exposed in the leg, ligatured, and then cut through just distal to the ligature. This effectively destroys many axons and leaves the proximal surviving component of the nerve cells. The surviving neurones are said to be 'axotomised.'

2. *Partial lesion of the sciatic nerve.* In this model, a ligature is passed through between one-third and one-half of the nerve in the upper third of the thigh. The ligature is pulled tight, which in effect transects the proportion of the nerve ligated. This model thus produces a 'partial' nerve injury (axotomy). Both this and the last model result in 'neuroma' formation at the site of transection.

3. *Spinal nerve transection model.* The nerve lesion in this model is produced nearer the spine. The procedure is essentially the same as the ligation and transection one described above. The lesion is produced in the ventral ramus of the spinal nerve before it unites with other rami to form the brachial, lumbar, or sacral plexuses. Experimental designs using rat L5 spinal nerve usually describe the nerve being 'transected and cut about 1–1.5 cm distal from the DRG' (e.g. Habler et al 2000). It is therefore not a nerve root lesion.

4. *Chronic constriction injury of the sciatic nerve.* Here, the sciatic nerve at mid thigh level is ligatured loosely to produce only a constriction effect. This light ligature causes the development of intraneural oedema whose swelling is prevented by the ligature and results in a 'self-strangulation' effect. This type of insult produces a degeneration, or interruption, in nearly all large myelinated and a great many of the smaller thinly myelinated Aδ fibres. A large percentage of unmyelinated (C fibres) afferents survive.

All four of these models of nerve injury lead to the animal exhibiting behavioural signs of pain—hence, they demonstrate autotomy or self-mutilation behaviour (Wall et al 1979), as well as signs of increased mechanical and thermal sensitivity in the territory of the injured nerve. The animals also show signs of ongoing pain, such as limping and guarding of the affected paw/limb, and develop some of the non-pain symptoms traditionally associated with RSD and causalgia. Hence, hypertrophic nail growth and abnormal skin temperature regulation, but swelling, even in the early stages is not seen and is therefore different to the situation seen in CRPS patients (Bennett & Roberts 1996).

But do the nerve injury models and the subsequent manipulation of the sympathetic nervous system prove that SMP exists? Bennett and Roberts (1996) are categorical: 'There is no question whatsoever that SMP exists in animals. In the partial and spinal nerve transection models sympathectomy or pharmacological sympathetic block appears to completely eliminate the abnormal pain sensations.' Also, '...the animal work has taught us that SMP is a real organic phenomenon' (pp. 115–116).

However, writing some five years later and reviewing the topic, Janig and Baron (2001) are more cautious about the interpretations of many of the experiments used to support the concept. They offer several warnings. For example:

- Not all laboratories agree with each others' findings—they cite many instances where conclusions do not concur and also offer alternative models and mechanisms for the effects noted.
- Small changes in experimental procedures can create major behavioural changes.
- In those experiments that manipulate the SNS using systemic pharmacological interventions, there may be widespread effects on a variety of other targets.
- Just as in humans, there may be significantly different mechanisms for quite similar symptoms between different individuals that have received the same injury. Just as some humans may be prone to developing post nerve injury CRPS with SMP or without it, so may different rats.
- The doses of pharmacological agents used to block or to stimulate the SNS in the experiments are frequently massive and unlikely to be 'physiological' (i.e. to occur naturally.)
- Surgical preparation of the animals can result in rapid changes in the expression of receptors and ionic channels so that longer-term abnormalities need to be interpreted with caution.
- Many observations made of *in-vitro* animal models do not match those of patients with SMP.

These observations and the authors' cautionary comments are certainly not to be taken as proof that SMP does not exist. What is clear is that sympathetic-afferent coupling can occur in pathophysiological conditions and that this does involve increased expression of adrenaline receptors on the lesioned afferent nerves as well as other 'plastic changes' in both the sympathetic and the afferent systems. Their warning is that the experimental interventions used seem out of proportion to biological events and hence should be interpreted with 'utmost caution'.

In their summary they conclude that:

1. Human models clearly show that the SNS is involved in pain and most likely produces associated tissue changes in patients with CRPS Type I and CRPS Type II.
2. Nerve lesions in animal models do alter the ongoing and reflex activity of the SNS and that a coupling between the SNS and the sensory system exists. This coupling has been found to occur, or may occur:
   - At the site of the nerve lesion.
   - Anywhere along the length of an unmyelinated nerve fibre that has regenerated to its target tissue following nerve injury.
   - In nociceptor fibre endings of intact cutaneous nerves whose nerve trunk has suffered a partial nerve injury.
   - Anywhere along the length of afferent nerve fibre axons proximal to the nerve injury.
   - In the dorsal root ganglion of injured nerves (see also, Michaelis 2000).
3. Many of the morphological changes observed in the nerve lesion models can be correlated with changes in function that may be relevant to SMP in CRPS Type -II, but not CRPS Type I.

As more and more experimental models wrestle with the problem there is an increasing recognition that the mechanisms are complex, multiple and changing even when the symptom picture remains relatively stable. For example, Habler et al (2000), investigating SMP using an animal model, assessed the effect of electrical stimulation of the lumbar sympathetic trunk and the application of noradrenaline on recorded activity of damaged (axotomised) afferents following L5 spinal nerve transection as described above. Surprisingly, they were unable to demonstrate excitatory behaviour in the majority of the nerves they stimulated at physiological levels, or applied noradrenaline to. In other words, there was no evidence of SMP. However, if the researchers first produced a vasoconstriction effect of the circulation to the L5 dorsal root ganglion, sympathetic stimulation did then produce a significant activation of the axotomised afferents. These researchers concluded that for a sympathetic-afferent coupling to occur following a spinal nerve transection injury, a significant vasoconstriction is required. A transient ischaemia may therefore be an important precondition for SMP in this region of the nerve.

As a clinical aside, or leap, it seems easy to envisage a situation of relative ischaemia in patients whose pain has led them to a situation of gross underactivity and very little cardiovascular load. Promoting immobility in the management of any condition walks hand in hand with the potential aggravating effects of ischaemia (see Chapter 2.) Immobility and the concomitant ischaemia that may occur could conceivably be a factor that predisposes to the development of sympathetic-afferent coupling and hence, SMP. Promoting or maintaining good circulation via regular action, exercise and normal movements in a way that, at least initially, avoids aggravating pain, may be an important preventative measure in the early management of nerve or tissue injury pain.

Models without nerve lesions

Bennett and Roberts (1996) rightly identified the need to explore the production of SMP in models without nerve damage in order to advance our understanding of CRPS Type I.

As noted in the previous chapter, early work has shown that the hyperalgesia which occurs in inflamed skin is made worse by noradrenaline and better by adrenoreceptor blockers and can be partially prevented by prior sympathectomy (see Levine et al 1986, Sato et al 1993). This C fibre noradrenaline sensitivity may be a normal physiological occurrence that disappears as inflammation subsides. Bennett and Roberts (1996) suggest that SMP would appear if either the inflammation persisted or the C-nociceptor noradrenaline responsiveness did not disappear with healing.

A further key finding of this work, also discussed in Chapter 3, is that skin nociceptor sensitisation that occurs as a result of experimental chemical irritation, requires the presence, but not the activity, of sympathetic terminals. The weight of the findings suggest that terminals act as a kind of docking station for the production of inflammatory agents like prostaglandins (see Levine et al 1986, Drummond 1995, Andreev et al 1995). This appears to offer further evidence that there is no requirement for sympathetic over-activity in the genesis of SMP in CRPS Type I. The physical presence of the sympathetic system seems to be an important factor.

Conclusions

Hopefully, many interesting points have emerged from this account and the evidence and discussions of the last two chapters. Here are a few that come to mind:

1. In CRPS there may or may not be SMP and it is impossible to tell whether it is present from the history or via physical testing.
2. In cases of CRPS with SMP there is little evidence for SNS over-activity in relation to pain; the current focus of attention is on abnormal adrenaline/noradrenaline sensitivity of the sensory/nociceptive system.
3. In CRPS, though still very unclear and poorly researched, there is a general assumption that changes in sympathetic activity may play a part in the development of non-pain symptoms like swelling, circulatory changes, oedema, temperature changes, sweating abnormalities and trophic dysfunction (see Chapter 2.) These changes may secondarily influence nociceptive sensitivity and activity (Janig 1996).
4. Sensory afferent nerve fibres can become maladaptively sensitive to the secretions of the SNS, i.e. to noradrenaline and adrenaline. This provides an efferent–afferent connection between the SNS and the nociceptive system that is not available in normal homeostatic conditions. It can thus

be seen as pathological/maladaptive. If there is some adaptive function provided by this injury-induced connection, no one has yet identified it or addressed its purpose.

5. There is a difference between animal models and patients in the behaviour and reproducibility of SMP.

6. Injury to different sites of the nervous system result in different mechanisms of pain and symptom production. For example, it seems that distally placed experimental nerve lesions, rather than proximal ones, are more likely to result in SMP.

7. Pain mechanisms change with time, often quite rapidly, even though the symptom picture may appear stable.

8. Simple answers based on simple constructs can be misleading and may lead to poorly reasoned and potentially harmful interventions.

9. The belief here is that CRPS and the SMP/SIP that are characteristic of it, are maladaptive symptoms in a maladaptive condition and as such *should* be preventable. Some individuals may be at risk to develop the condition.

10. Thinking and reasoning that is confined to peripheral tissues and nerves is untenable. Complex pain states involve all levels of the nervous system—input systems, scrutinising systems, and output systems. All models of understanding must include psychological and environmental factors.

11. Greater knowledge of mechanisms of pain, like those described here and in previous chapters and volumes should add to our profession's knowledge base and provide us all with an increased confidence. Patients should be the beneficiaries.

12. Physiotherapists have an important role to play in the continued development of the understanding of pain. Unbiased clinical observations may be particularly important. Most descriptions of diseases, syndromes, and disorders are derived from long out-of-date texts or standard textbooks that rely on observations of patients recorded a great many years ago and which have not been subjected to serious scrutiny. What patients feel and what clinicians think the patient feels may be quite different.

This chapter has outlined the evidence and controversies surrounding the concept of sympathetically maintained pain. The evidence suggests that there is value to this concept; but what constitutes it remains in need of further clarification.

REFERENCES

Ali Z, Raja SN, Wesselmann U, Fuchs PN, Meyer RA, Campbell JN 2000 Intradermal injection of norepinephrine evokes pain in patients with sympathetically maintained pain. Pain 88:161–168

Andreev NY, Dimitrevia N, Koltzenberg M, McMahon SB 1995 Peripheral administration of nerve growth factor in the adult rat produces a thermal hyperalgesia that requires the presence of sympathetic postganglionic neurones. Pain 63:109–115

Baron R, Wasner G, Borgstedt R, Hastedt E, Schulte H, Binder A, Kopper F, Rowbotham M, Levine JD, Fields HL 1999 Effect of sympathetic activity on capsaicin evoked pain, hyperalgesia, and vasodilation. Neurology 52:923–932

Baron R, Levine JD, Fields HL 1999a Causalgia and reflex sympathetic dystrophy. Does the sympathetic nervous system contribute to the generation of pain. Muscle and Nerve 22:678–695

Bennett GJ 1999 Scientific basis for the evaluation and treatment of RSD/CRPS syndromes: laboratory studies in animals and man. In: Max M (ed) Pain 1999—an updated review. IASP Press, Seattle

Bennett GJ, Roberts WJ 1996 Animal models and their contribution to our understanding of complex regional pain syndrome I and II. In: Janig W, Stanton-Hicks M (eds) Reflex Sympathetic Dystrophy: A Reappraisal. IASP Press, Seattle

Black JA, Dib-Hajj S, Cummins TR et al 2001 Sodium channels as therapeutic targets in neuropathic pain. In: Hansson PT, Fields H, Hill RG et al (eds) Neuropathic Pain: Pathophysiology and Treatment, Progress in Pain Research and Management, Vol 21. IASP Press, Seattle 19–36

Campbell JN, Meyer RA, Raja SN 1992 Is nociceptor activation by alpha-1 adrenoreceptors the culprit in sympathetically maintained pain? American Pain Society Journal 1:3–11

Campbell JN, Raja SN, Selig DK, Belzberg AJ, Meyer RA 1994 Diagnosis and management of sympathetically maintained pain. In: Fields HF, Liebeskind JC (eds) Pharmacological Approaches to the Treatment of Chronic Pain: New concepts and clinical issues. IASP Press, Seattle

Cepeda MS 1995 Autonomic nervous system and pain. Current Opinion in Anaesthesiology 8:450–454

Dotson R 1993 Causalgia—Reflex sympathetic dystrophy—sympathetically maintained pain: myth and reality. Muscle and Nerve 16:1049–1055

Drummond PD 1995 Noradrenaline increases hyperalgesia to heat in skin sensitised by capsaicin. Pain 60:311–315

Glynn CJ, Stannard C, Collins PA, Casale R 1993 The role of peripheral sudomotor blockade in the treatment of patients with sympathetically maintained pain. Pain 53: 39–42

Habler HJ, Eschenfelder S, Liu X-G, Janig W 2000 Sympathetic-sensory coupling after l5 spinal nerve lesion in the rat and its changes in dorsal root ganglion blood flow. Pain 87:335–345

Hannington-Kiff J 1974 Intravenous regional sympathetic blockade. Lancet 1: 1919–1920

Janig W 1992 Can reflex sympathetic dystrophy be reduced to an alpha-adrenoreceptor disease? American Pain Society Journal 1 (1): 16–22

Janig W 1996 The puzzle of 'reflex sympathetic dystrophy': mechanisms, hypothesis, open questions In: Janig W, Stanton-Hicks M (eds) Reflex Sympathetic Dystrophy: A reappraisal. IASP Press, Seattle

Janig W, Baron R 2001 The role of the sympathetic nervous system in neuropathic pain: Clinical observations and animal models. In: Hansson PT, Fields HL, Hill RG et al (eds) Neuropathic Pain: Pathophysiology and treatment. Progress in pain research and management Vol 21. IASP Press, Seattle 125–149

Kingery WS 1997 A critical review of controlled clinical trials for peripheral neuropathic pain and complex regional pain syndromes. Pain 73: 123–139

Kramis RC, Roberts WJ, Gillette RG 1996 Post sympathectomy neuralgia: hypothesis on peripheral and central mechanisms. Pain 64: 1–9

Levine JD, Taiwo YO, Collins SD, Tam JK 1986 Noradrenaline hyperalgesia is mediated through interaction with sympathetic postganglionic neurone terminals rather than activation of primary afferent nociceptors. Nature 323:158–160

Livingstone WK 1943 Pain Mechanism. Macmillan New York

Max MB, Gilron I 1999 Sympathetically maintained pain: Has the emperor no clothes? Neurology 52:905–907

McQuay H, Moore A 1998 An Evidence-based Resource For Pain Relief. Oxford University Press, Oxford

Michaelis M 2000 Coupling of sympathetic and somatosensory neurons following nerve injury: Mechanisms and potential significance for the generation of pain. In: Devor M, Rowbotham MC, Wiesenfeld-Hallin Z (eds) Proceedings of the 9th World Congress on Pain, Progress in Pain Research and Management, Vol 16. IASP Press, Seattle 645–656

Noon M 2002 Placebo and the therapeutic alliance. In: Gifford LS (ed) Topical Issues in Pain 4. Placebo and nocebo. Muscles and Pain. Pain Management. CNS Press, Falmouth

Perl ER 1994 A reevaluation of mechanisms leading to sympathetically related pain. In: Fields HF, Liebeskind JC (eds) Pharmacological approaches to the treatment of chronic pain: New concepts and clinical issues. IASP Press, Seattle

Price DD, Gracely RH, Bennett GJ 1996 The challenge and the problem of placebo in assessment of sympathetically maintained pain. In: Janig W, Stanton-Hicks (eds) Reflex Sympathetic Dystrophy: A reappraisal. IASP Press, Seattle

Price DD, Long S, Wilsey B, Rafii A 1998 Analysis of peak duration of analgesia produced by local anaesthetic injected into sympathetic ganglia of complex regional pain syndrome patients. The Clinical Journal of Pain 14:216–226

Ramamurthy S Hoffman J 1995 Intavenous regional guanethidine in the treatment of reflex sympathetic dystrophy/causalgia: a randomised, double-blind study. Anaesthesia and Analgesia 81: 718–723

Roberts WJ 1986 A hypothesis on the physiological basis for causalgia and related pains. Pain 24:297–311

Sato J, Suzuki S, Iseki T, Kumazawa T 1993 Adrenergic excitation of cutaneous nociceptors in chronically inflamed rats . Neuroscience Letters 164:225–228

Scadding JW 1999 Complex regional pain syndrome. In: Wall PD, Melzack R (eds) The Textbook of Pain 4th edn Chruchill Livingstone, Edinburgh 835–849

Schwartzman RJ, McClellan TL 1987 Reflex sympathetic dystrophy: A review. Archives of Neurology 44:555

Shortall R 2002 The powerful placebo—hit or myth? In: Gifford LS (ed) Topical Issues in Pain 4. Placebo and nocebo. Muscles and Pain. Pain Management. CNS Press, Falmouth

Thompson SWN 2001 Is the sympathetic nervous system a pain? Neuroscience News 4 (3): 35–41

Torebjork E, Wahren L, Wallin G, Halling R, Koltzenburg M 1995 Noradrenaline-evoked pain in neuralgia. Pain 63:11–20

Walker AE, Nulson F 1948 Electrical stimulation of the upper thoracic portion of the sympathetic chain in man. Archives of Neurology and Psychiatry 59:559–560

Wall PD 1995 Noradrenaline-evoked pain in neuralgia. Pain 63: 1–2

Wall PD 1999 Personal communication

Wall PD, Gutnik M 1974 Ongoing activity in peripheral nerves: The physiology and pharmacology of impulses originating from a neuroma. Experimantal Neurology 43:580–593

Wall PD, Gutnik M 1974a properties of afferent nerve impulse from a neuroma. Nature 248:740–743

Wall PD, Devor M, Inbal R 1979 Autotomy following peripheral nerve lesions: experimental anaesthesia dolorosa. Pain 7:103–113

White JC, Sweet WH 1969 Pain and the Neurosurgeon: A forty year experience. C C Thomas, Springfield

Wynn-Parry CB 1996 Rehabilitation of reflex sympathetic dystrophy. Clinical Orthopaedics 1, (2): 327–338

5

A review of physiotherapy management of complex regional pain syndrome

MICK THACKER AND LOUIS GIFFORD

Introduction

The physiotherapy management of CRPS mirrors that of most conditions, i.e. although widely advocated there is little in the way of strong scientific evidence to support the use of our interventions. Nearly all the major medical experts in this field advocate the use of physiotherapy but seldom offer much more than a few passing words or a list of techniques. While physiotherapy is supported, a key question is—do we really know what we are doing, or should be doing, with this condition?

Reviewing the physiotherapy literature leaves one realising that there is very little that hasn't been tried. Though not strongly supported by treatment trials, it is likely that modality based therapies as well as activation approaches are of some benefit in this complex and disabling condition. What has been encouraging in the last few years is the recognition of the multifaceted nature of the condition and hence the need for a multifaceted, multidimensional and multidisciplinary management approach. As will be discussed, more rational and better guidelines for therapy are evolving and being published (see Stanton-Hicks et al 1998).

This chapter will review the literature that relates to the management of CRPS in the adult population. There is also a detailed discussion of the implications of the review findings for the formulation of better management strategies.

Historical perspective

The management of this painful condition has been characterised by an approach that was at best aggressive and at worst torture! My (Thacker) own earliest clinical guidance for treatment of this condition was to be told that I must move the affected hand or foot no matter what the patient felt or complained of. Although one could object to what is basically a semantic discussion, the word *aggressive* is noted repeatedly in the literature in relation to the prescription for physiotherapy. We much prefer the term *proactive*. This aims to develop a forward thinking, patient driven and centered, active approach to therapy which attempts to overcome the negative and frightening physical connotations that are the undoubted legacy of the word aggressive.

Other noticeable aspects of therapy have been the general acceptance that there is some form of sympathetic over-activity/abnormality dominating the presentation of the patient. Many of the interventions proposed over the years have been specifically targeted at such 'over-activity.' Apparent successes reported by advocates of such approaches are often used as evidence to lend support to the concept that the sympathetic nervous system (SNS) is faulty/overactive/blameworthy, thus perpetuating the outdated concept of abnormally increased sympathetic tone (see discussion in previous chapters.)

A further observation arising from a survey of the literature is that the management of pain in CRPS patients is often dealt with medically and within a strict medical model. Also, as a generalisation, most physiotherapy approaches to pain relief focus on TENS and/or acupuncture (but see below.) Is it possible that we have forgotten the therapeutic value of carefully prescribed active movement as an analgesic in these patients? (The reader is advised to consult an excellent paper by Harding, 1999.)

Lastly many accounts prescribe therapy dependent on the stage of the disorder. This is an outdated concept (see Stanton Hicks et al 1995 and Chapter 2.) Current thinking, and the advice suggested here, is that treatment selection should be patient and problem specific rather than reliant on challengeable pathological or theoretical constructs that many now believe to be floored (Stanton Hicks et al 1998).

Review of modalities reported for the treatment of RSD/Causalgia (CRPS Types I and II)

Electrotherapy

There is a lack of detailed information in the majority of studies looking at specific electrotherapy modalities. The following is therefore a necessarily brief discussion of relevant material.

TENS

TENS is the most quoted non-pharmacological modality for pain relief in this condition. Unfortunately, there is little in the way of high quality evidence to support its use. Papers detailing successful pain relief from TENS in CRPS are almost exclusively single case studies with little guidance on dosage (Fitzpatrick 2000, Thomas 1996). A literature search in April, 2002, revealed only three papers when combining the terms reflex sympathetic dystrophy, complex regional pain syndrome, and TENS.

This leads to obvious problems for the practising clinician who is seeking guidance over treatment selection and application. Extrapolation from successful regimens used for other neuropathic and ongoing pain states may be reasonable, since many of the clinical presentations and underlying mechanisms are similar.

Since the mature literature on CRPS is now more questioning and cautious regarding cause, a degree of care is required where treatment selection and dosage is based on rigid pathological models or dogmatic statements in texts and papers. Some knowledge of underlying pain mechanisms can help in decision making, though. For instance, we now know that pain mechanisms alter and change as time goes on (see previous chapters.) This may help give better explanations for some of the difficulties encountered in treatment choice as well as provide reasons why some patients may respond better than others. Also, TENS settings that excite large myelinated Aβ fibres (i.e. high frequency settings but often low settings too), may, in individuals with mechanically evoked allodynia (extreme hypersensitivity to touch or movement), cause extreme exacerbation of symptoms. Since it is known that central sensitisation (Chapter 3) allows Aβ fibre input to access nociceptor pathways and hence cause pain, this phenomenon can be understood easily. One requirement for successful TENS application in patients exhibiting this high sensitivity response might be for the therapist and patient to search for areas of electrode placement that are beneficial, or better still that can be used in an incremental way to bring about progressive desensitisation. This implies things like graded increases of current as well as progression of electrode placement into areas of heightened sensitivity and reactivity if at all possible.

It is often the case that this type of TENS hypersensitivity is a dominant feature in one patient whilst completely absent in another. Although Walker and Cousins (1996) have warned of the potential for negative effects of TENS in CRPS patients, this should not deter therapists from using it if changes in application can be made so that progress in sensitivity control or pain management are achieved.

There are several references to the effects of electrostimulatory modalities on blood flow with a proposal of some effect on vasomotor activity (e.g. Low 1994). This has been suggested to be of potential benefit to patients with CRPS. A warning is that while TENS may alter vasomotor activity, the reasoning to support its use relies on an exclusively peripheral mechanism based model that assumes sympathetic nervous system dysfunction requiring correction.

Hardy and Hardy (1997) attempt a more objective approach to the use of TENS effects. They highlight its potential influence on temperature control (generally accepted as an indicator of vasomotor activity) and suggest that, with careful monitoring of temperature together with the patient's subjective responses, it may be possible for clinicians to bias the TENS effect towards stimulation on blood flow if required.

It is important to recognise that successful use of TENS does not reliably indicate that any *specific* analgesic mechanism is operating. Within a patient we know that all forms and applications of TENS have widespread modes of action at many levels. For example, as in all therapies, there are likely to be effects determined via psychophysiologically activated pathways (see the Lawes chapter in Volume 4 of this series.)

Barbara Headley supported the use of TENS for CRPS patients back in the late 1980s (Headly 1987). She described how the exact mode of action of TENS in general and more specifically in CRPS was unknown. She intimated that a better understanding of the mechanism of action of TENS would result in a more rational decision over the settings used and the overall treatment protocol. The evidence available to date suggests that this has not yet occurred!

Taylor-Mullins (1989) stated that TENS (high frequency) would not by itself alleviate all the pain associated with CRPS but proposed that it may produce enough relief to facilitate other interventions, a theme supported by others (Headley 1987, Hardy and Hardy 1997, Thomas 1996, Stanton Hicks 1998).

Fredorczyk (1997) reported that there was a paucity of studies to support the use of TENS in painful conditions of the upper extremity.

Withrington and Wynn Parry (1984) offer a useful observation on TENS: 'This is an extremely valuable, but much abused modality of treatment. Far too often pain clinics hand the patient a stimulator with only the briefest instructions of how to use it, and not surprisingly the treatment proves ineffective.' They suggest that before discarding the modality several parameters including pulse width, repetition and pattern, electrode placement and duration of use should be experimented with.

An important aspect to the use of TENS is that whilst it is seemingly a passive therapy, it can be viewed as an active therapy in that it involves patients in their own management and as such offers a means of their having at least some control. This effect may be intensified if the individual understands its principles and is allowed to be actively engaged in a trial and error approach to find the most effective settings and mode of application.

Although Hareau (1996) strongly advocates the use of TENS in the management of pain in patients with CPRS, she suggests that it should be discontinued if it appears that the patient is becoming dependent on the modality. Unfortunately she fails to offer any help in how to identify potential 'TENS junkies' or a pathway of management to help patients reduce their dependency.

Interferential therapy

Some common texts claim that the autonomic nervous system can be manipulated using this modality (Low & Reed 1994, Savage 1984). It is interesting to note that the more scientific the text, the less likely it is that such claims are found (Martin 1996). There is no convincing evidence in the literature searched that this therapy can alter either sympathetic or parasympathetic activity. However, it is worth reasoning that the way in which an individual reacts to the treatment stimulus may have a bearing on their autonomic tone.

Ultrasound

In discussing the use of ultrasound in the management of CRPS most authors refer to a paper by Portwood et al (1987). The paper offers three case studies to support tenuous claims of positive outcomes noted in their patients. There are no controls and all three patients received other interventions, too.

Harden (2000) stated that ultrasound was less effective in his clinic compared with the results of Portwood et al (1987). Unfortunately Harden's work has some methodological flaws; for example he fails to give the number of subjects from which he obtained his data.

At a mechanistic and purely peripheral level of reasoning, the use of ultrasound can be questioned since its effects are reported to be 'pro' inflammatory. As CRPS is thought to involve exaggeration/recruitment of the inflammatory and/or immune responses (see Chapters 2 & 3) this type of effect may be provocative.

Biofeedback

Grunert et al (1990) reported positive results when using thermal biofeedback (combined with relaxation and psychotherapy) in a group of individuals with residual RSD (CRPS Type I). They studied a group of 20 patients who had histories of repeated poor responses to other interventions. They used both visual and audible biofeedback to teach patients how to control their peripheral blood flow. They allowed patients to use the device during activities of daily living and relaxation. Their outcomes showed that the patients were able to learn how to control their blood flow as well as demonstrate a significant reduction in pain which was still present at a follow up 12 months later.

This study is limited by the usual criticisms of no control group and multiple interventions. However, the total package of care does demonstrate the desirable effects which occur *when patients are given some form of control and involvement in their own management.* This in itself could account for the alterations in blood flow noted as there would be a change in the SNS due to alterations in psychological driving mechanisms.

Hardy and Hardy (1997) advocated the use of thermal biofeedback although the only source they quoted to support the inclusion of this modality into their therapeutic regimen was the Grunert et al (1990) paper.

Earlier Headley (1987) discussed biofeedback as a potential intervention in the management of RSD (CRPS Type I). She cited the work from two papers (Blanchard 1979, Fischer-Williams et al 1981) that reported positive preliminary results in patients with RSD. What is interesting to observe is that the case studies presented in these papers show a degree of commonality with the work of Grunert et al (1990) in that the responders had proved refractory to other therapies. Apart from the important 'control' aspect mentioned, it may be that newly introduced therapies, enthusiastically offered, have a 'novelty factor' effect that in some way kick starts positive biological responses. Here again, psychologically initiated and recruited mechanisms may underpin the positive changes observed.

Muscle stimulation

There are some advocates of the use of electrical stimulation of muscles in patients with CRPS Type I (Hareau 1996, Thomas 1996). As with other modalities there is no good trial evidence offered to support the use of these interventions. The suggested aims for such interventions include increasing blood flow, mobilising stiff joints, and increasing the strength of the musculo-tendinous apparatus (Hareau 1996, Thomas 1996).

Taylor-Mullins (1989) proposed the use of electrical muscle stimulation combined with compression bandaging to reduce the oedema associated with CRPS.

Iontophoresis

The transdermal application of guanethidine was first suggested by Hannington-Kiff in the mid-1980s. The treatment application followed observed successes with the drug when injected to produce a regional blockade (Hannington-Kiff 1984, see Chapter 4). The delivery of a drug using iontophoresis is dependent on its charge when in solution. Fortunately guanethidine has a high positive charge and therefore is relatively easy to deliver in this way.

Hannington-Kiff (1984) like most others, used a few non-controlled case studies to support the positive role of this blocking procedure. He reported that the individuals receiving the therapy gained immediate pain relief from the intervention. This observation raises interest since guanethidine blocks normally evoke an immediate *increase* in sympathetically maintained pain due to the massive initial noradrenaline release that it produces in the tissues (see Chapter 4.) It is of course possible that the individuals treated lacked adrenosensitivity in the tissues that the drug reached, or that transdermal application of the drug has a different mode of action. Sound reasoning for the effect should always include non-specific therapeutic effects (see placebo chapters in Volume 4) as well as the possibility that the current generated to produce the iontophoresis may have had a role to play too!

Heating

Warming the tissues has been advocated in the management of CRPS both to desensitise the tissues and to induce some pain relief (Charlton 1991,

Hareau 1996, Lampen-Smith 1997, Fredorczyk 1997, Stanton Hicks et al 1998, Harden 2000). The majority of these authors do not recommend any particular method of producing therapeutic heating. Whilst there is little 'scientific' evidence to support the use of heat, as we all know, many patients report that it is effective in providing a temporary reduction in pain.

Acupuncture

Ernst et al's (1995) paper is one of the few reports of this modality in the management of CPRS Type I. They demonstrated a reduction in pain, measured using a visual analogue scale, between a group receiving traditional Chinese acupuncture and a group receiving a sham procedure. Unfortunately the title of this article is somewhat deceptive as it leads one to think that they conducted a large scale randomised control trial (RCT—see Chapters 9 & 10). In fact they investigated only 14 patients and failed to use any statistical tests to analyse their results. The sham procedure, far from being physiologically inactive, involved the needling of the tissue at 'non acupuncture' points. It is important for clinicians to be aware that a great many studies have shown equal therapeutic effects whether needling is performed on recognised acupuncture points or not (see Melzack 1994).

Scrutiny of the results of Ernst et al (1995) also revealed a large degree of variance at each data point (indicted by large overlapping error bars on the graphs). Results like these, that lack a proper statistical analysis, should leave the reader with serious doubts about the validity of the claim that traditional acupuncture is a globally effective modality in the relief of pain in CRPS Type I.

There are a couple of dated studies (Chan & Chow 1981, Leo 1983) that have attempted to ascertain the benefit of electro-acupuncture in the management of this condition, but they have serious methodological flaws and are therefore of dubious value in terms of clarifying the situation. (See also Lesley Smith's analysis in Chapter 10.)

Splinting

Splinting was widely advocated in the older literature on CRPS Type I (Headley 1987, Taylor-Mullins 1989). Unsurprisingly, there has been little evidence to support its use. Even so, this modality still has some protagonists. For example, Thomas (1996) advocates the use of splinting (both resting and functional) in the management of those with upper limb CRPS Type I. His support is based solely on his own clinical observations. Most specialist hand and plastic surgery departments still suggest that splinting may be useful if used in conjunction with an active rehabilitation program (personal communication J. Leathwood, London.)

A review of the discussion on immobility in Chapter 2 highlights the potential harm that may be caused by injudicious splinting and casting that reinforces the patients' unwillingness to move.

Desensitisation

Most authors include some sort of desensitisation program as part of overall patient management (Headley 1987, Hareau 1996, Fitzpatrick 2000). Hardy and Hardy (1997) give sensible advice on desensitisation of hypersensitivities relating to vibration, touch, heat and cold . This is one approach that has some evidence to support its use and the reader is referred to consult their work as a resource (see also Chapter 6.)

Harden (2000) supports the use of desensitisation strategies and suggests that as well as specific techniques like those above, general exercise itself may act as a desensitiser of the person as a whole, perhaps reducing the maladaptive high 'gain' of their nervous system.

Movement and CRPS

The literature suggesting that movement is an essential component in the management of CRPS would pretty much include the whole of the reference list cited at the end of this chapter. This overwhelming support is based almost exclusively on clinical observation or relates to the simple fact that these patients are so often not moving and need to in order to have some sort of life.

Although there are no RCTs that look specifically at the use of movement based therapies in the management of this condition, there remains a firm consensus of opinion that movement based therapies should be *aggressive or vigorous*. Thankfully, Thomas (1996) rightly points out that such an approach may lead to a breakdown in patient confidence and reluctance on the part of patients to participate fully in their therapy. Overcoming the common chronic pain scenario, whereby the patient lurches from periods of overactivity and flare up to prolonged underactivity/rest, by careful planning, pacing and graded increases in activity are now well established and should be taken on here (see other management chapters in these volumes; also, Main & Spanswick 2000).

The movement based therapies that have been advocated range from passive mobilisations right through to self directed techniques aimed at compressing the joint surfaces. A frequent suggestion is for progress to move from passive through to active movement being often linked to the determined staging of the disorder. There are however more structured approaches to therapy such as the 'Scrub and Carry' regimen of Carlson and Watson (1988) (see below.)

In a recent highly recommended article, Stanton Hicks et al (1998) proposed guidelines for CRPS management that included various movement based strategies. Whilst unsubstantiated by any large clinical trial the progressive multilevel and multidisciplinary management approach is one which is now universally accepted for any ongoing pain state. A key focus of the approach is that of functional restoration. Here, all interventions, as far as possible, work together and are geared to promoting the achievement of time dependent goals.

The term kinesiaphobic has been used (Boas 1999; Vlaeyen & Linton 2000) to describe the observation that most patients with severe and long standing pain disorders have a dislike of movement if not an intense fear of it (see the section on fear avoidance, Volume 1 of this series.) Therapists are advised to respect such feelings. Patient fear of movement may be based on the experience of the provocation of intense pain or the belief that they may experience pain with a given movement. They may also fear further damage. The use of overtly aggressive or rigorous techniques and approaches is likely not only to be highly unproductive but also to promote further fear and anxiety of movement and result in increased disability (Vlaeyen & Linton 2000).

For this review, movement techniques have been split into the following categories: passive mobilisations, massage, and active exercises. Functional restoration and progressive loading are also discussed at the end of this chapter.

Passive mobilisations

All types of passive movements have been advocated to maintain/increase range of movement in CRPS patients. Hardy and Hardy (1997) advocated the use of continuous passive movement with the suggestion that it would allow pain free movement when hands-on approaches increase pain. This is a commonly recommended but un-researched modality (Taylor-Mullins 1989, Hareau 1996, Harden 2000).

A mechanistic and mechanism-based manual therapy reasoning approach has led to the application of 'targeted' passive mobilisation techniques for the management of 'sympathetic components' of disorders like CRPS. The techniques include, cervical side gliding, sympathetic slumping, and thoracic mobilisation.

Through the 1990s Wright, Slater and Vincenzino have been responsible for much of the work and interest in the effect of passive manual therapies on peripheral SNS activity (Slater 1995; Slater et al 1993,1994; Vincenzino et al 1994, 1998, 1999). Recently, Slater (2001) has pointed out that reproduction of symptoms by the sympathetic slump does not indicate that the SNS is involved in the condition, but more likely that the nervous system as a whole is sensitive to movement.

The work of Wright, Slater and Vincenzino noted above, suggests that there is a period of sympathetic excitation following the manoeuvers listed above and it is this finding that has led them to speculate on the mechanisms behind post manipulative pain relief. Others however have voiced caution and offered different interpretations and opinions (Zusman 1995, Thacker 1995). This work will be discussed in more detail in a later section.

The variable response of the SNS when measured following a high velocity thrust manipulation has been studied (Larson et al 1980, Kappler & Kelso 1984, Harris & Wagnon 1987). Both inhibitory and excitatory effects have been shown in normal subjects and those with symptoms/pathologies. Closer inspection of this work highlights several methodological flaws, most notably the lack of suitable controls and the methods of monitoring changes in blood flow and skin conductance. It is interesting to note that the osteopathic and chiropractic professions seem to have moved away from using sympathetically mediated mechanisms to explain the effects of manipulation.

Clinicians need to be alert to the fact that touch alone has been shown to alter sympathetic activity (Appenzeller 1990). This suggests that there is an important need for an appropriate control group if the true effect of different manual interventions are to be fully described and understood.

As far as the SNS is concerned it may be well worth considering touch, manual therapy, mobilisations, or manipulations (or any therapy for that matter) on a spectrum of 'perceived threat' for a given patient. Thus, it would be predicted that a technique rated as a high 'threat' would strongly activate the SNS whilst those who perceive a technique more positively / of low threat, are likely to have only a modest sympathetic activation. Consider also that patients' perception of what is being done to them is likely to change from one moment to the next and therefore may be reflected in their sympathetic activity (Gifford 1998). If this is indeed the case, and the desire is to avoid a 'sympathetic' response, it supports the need for adequate preparation / advice / explanation of an intervention or technique before it is performed. On the other hand, and not recommended, if a high sympathetic response is deemed desirable, then it may be best to maintain an air of mystery, novelty, fear and the unexpected!

Massage

Although not strictly a movement based therapy, massage is often discussed with other manual therapies. Various massage techniques have been proposed as useful interventions in the management of CRPS Type I. Lampen-Smith (1997) has suggested that the main aim of massage interventions is to increase blood flow / venous return, encourage lymphatic drainage and to aid in the relief of pain. She offers a reasonable level of support for the use of massage in CRPS Type I patients. This is of interest when compared with the lack of references to support other interventions.

Frazer (1978) published a single case study demonstrating a positive response to connective tissue massage with a CRPS Type I patient. Unfortunately the presentation suffers from many problems associated with case studies of its era and so does not allow us to extrapolate.

One observation is that therapies such as massage may be, on the one hand, just as effective as other passive manual therapies, and on the other far less complicated and far easier and quicker to learn. Massage can also be easily done by the patient or spouses / relations and be seen as an active part of a graded, desensitising programme along side other management processes.

Comment on passive therapy approaches

The difficulties in decision making faced by hands-on passive management is highlighted when approaches to patients with upper limb CRPS by manual therapists are compared to those advocated by specialist hand therapists. For 'peripheral' symptoms manual therapists might prioritise treatments that attend to spinal sources, or 'comparable spinal signs' found via physical assessment. Findings may in turn be linked to constructs of sympathetic involvement relating to issues like pathomechanics of the sympathetic chain or to 'facilitated segments' at appropriate levels. One hypothesis seems to be that therapy directed towards the spine and/or the sympathetic trunk may impact sympathetic activity in a beneficial direction (see discussion in Section 1). The hand therapist meanwhile concentrates efforts in the peripheral tissues, integrating mobilisation techniques of selected hypersenstive and/or hypomobile tissues along side progressive functional challenge.

Luckily, therapists have a certain freedom to operate in a trial and error fashion in order to bring about progress that is very often governed by the patient's pain response. What is evident is that constructs that relate the clinical presentation and the treatment approach to a particular mechanism are often very useful in justifying a novel approach. This is particularly so when a problem is well known for being difficult to help, combined with a form of therapy which might appear a little far fetched.

It is always worth considering what the patient might be thinking. Thus, justification is particularly important for the patient who could well find treatments of the spine, in sometimes very contorted positions, quite difficult to accept or to see as relevant. After all, it is hard to *believe* in something (an important requirement of the placebo response) if we do not understand it in the first place! Therapists using techniques whose focus of approach is on the spine for distal symptoms might be well advised to spend time explaining their underlying rationale (see placebo chapters in Volume 4).

Perhaps the most important point is to advise that therapists try to avoid getting carried away with the apparent power behind complicated manual therapy techniques and consider the technique as just one possibility, or more bluntly, a modest and questionable 'modality' in a management programme whose major aim is functional restoration and physical confidence.

The idea that pain relief has to be achieved before functional recovery is likely to be unproductive and unfulfilling. Time and again predominantly passive pain focused approaches are being criticised in chapters and essays, like those found in this and the other volumes in this series, as well as in the mature literature on chronic pain prevention and management. Readers are particularly alerted to the frequent statement that *passive therapy* with *high expectations* of pain relief/cure/fix, whether provided by hands, machines or tablets, may be making the patient become *reliant* on the therapy, pain fixated, fearful of movement and unnecessarily shifted towards a passive style of coping. Factors like these are seen as significant factors in causing rather than preventing chronic incapacity.

Active exercise

It makes logical sense to promote active movement and function in an individual who has limited function, limited ranges of movement and significant fear of movement and its consequences (see Volume 1 of this series.) It is therefore unsurprising that the use of active movement as a part of management programs is now so widely advocated (Charlton 1991, Hareau 1996, Lampen-Smith 1997, Stanton Hicks 1998, Stanton Hicks et al 1998, Harding 1999, Fitzpatrick 2000). All these authors suggest the biggest obstacle to the restoration of movement is the presence and impact of pain.

Various exercises and concepts have been proposed to help restore active movement but perhaps the most widely advocated for CRPS is the 'Scrub and Carry' regimen of Watson and Carlson (Watson & Carlson 1987, Carlson & Watson 1988, Charlton 1991, Hardy & Hardy 1997, Stanton Hicks 1998). This involves a progressive pattern of axial loading (compression) and distraction. This program has received support as it is thought not only to encourage movement but also to help desensitise the affected extremity. The name comes from the original authors use of a scrubbing brush to facilitate vertical compression of the limb and the use of a brief case / bag to provide a load to provide axial distraction! In line with other desensitising and activating programmes they advocated a build up (graded exposure) of these forces over time. However, even though the regimen is now quite old there is as yet no good evidence for its widespread support.

Hareau (1996) advocates an exercise approach that works from proximal to distal which has obvious parallels with the management of neurological conditions. Hareau (1996) suggests that the approach minimises the chance of exacerbation of the patient's symptoms.

Discussion 1: Manual therapy, sympathetic effects and the sympathetic slump

It is the opinion here that we are at a cross-roads in the professional development of physiotherapy. On the one hand we desire better and more scientific evidence and explanations for our interventions, while on the other we are uncomfortable and uneasy with what we may find.

Mention was made earlier of the work that has focused on manual therapy induced SNS change and an extended discussion of this work is presented here.

This work, and its clinical interpretations, seems to have had a powerful, almost global, impact on manual therapy approaches to pain and its relation to conditions that traditionally contain 'sympathetically labelled' phenomena. Since closer scrutiny of the work reveals some potential challenges and flaws with the results and their interpretations, I (Thacker) feel it important and appropriate to outline them here. It is desirable that this discussion is seen not as unnecessary intellectual niggling but as part of the important process of mature scientific appraisal whose goal is ultimately the good of the patient and the standing of the physiotherapy profession.

Slater (1991) hypothesised that a modified version of the slump test could be used to investigate the response of the sympathetic trunk to physical loading. Based on analysis of the anatomy and relations of the sympathetic trunk (see Chapter 1) in relation to spinal axes of movement and known nervous system dynamics, she proposed that a combination of movements could physically tension the ipsilateral sympathetic chain and ganglia. (To tension the right sympathetic chain the movements required are: in a long sitting position, add, thoracic spine flexion, side flexion and rotation to the left with cervical extension and left side flexion.)

Together with co-workers, Slater (Slater et al 1993, 1994) went on to investigate the effects of the 'sympathetic slump' combined with a rib mobilisation technique on a group of normal subjects. They were able to show that there was a slightly greater increase in skin conductance (due to increased sweating, see below), in the upper limbs in their experimental group, than in either a placebo condition or control group. They showed that although this effect was bilateral it was greater on the side of the loaded sympathetic chain. They also measured skin temperature and although the placebo and test results were significant versus the control [temperature was seen to decrease] they were not different from one another. They concluded that the sympathetic slump had excitatory physiological effects on the peripheral SNS function.

Further studies were performed using a neural tension test to load the upper limb nerve trunks and similar results were obtained. Again skin conductance was increased with no change in temperature versus placebo and control. Slater (1995) also published a study into the effects of the 'sympathetic slump' on a group of patients with frozen shoulder. Her results showed similar measurable effects to those of normal subjects quoted above, that is, an apparent sympathetic excitation. She concluded, with notable caution, that sympathetic slump alone was not likely to help in the treatment of patients with this condition.

Peterson et al (1993) showed that a grade III passive mobilisation technique applied to the C5 vertebra increased sympathetic activity in the upper limbs of normal subjects. They monitored both temperature (as a measure of vasomotor activity) and skin conductance (sudomotor function) and included a placebo condition in the trial. They suggested that these responses might underlie the analgesic effect of mobilisation techniques.

The results and conclusions of these investigations are open to alternative interpretations.

All of the above studies used direct measurement of skin conductance in the upper limb as a determinant of the sympathetic response to the physical testing procedures. (Skin conductance is a measure of sweat production/ sudomotor function: increased moisture on the skin leads to a lower impedance of the skin.) They all reported significant increases in their experimental and placebo groups with increases also noted between these groups in a pattern in favour of the treatment groups.

One criticism is that they tested sudomotor function (skin conductance) in each case over the palmar aspect of the thumb and/or index fingers. While this seems straight forward, it is known that sudomotor activity of the sweat glands on the palmar aspect of the hand are controlled solely by the psycho-emotional centres (personal experience of sweaty palms associated with nerves supports this!) and though reflexogenically mediated via the sympathetic efferents to the palm, may really represent a measure of the psycho-emotional drive (Appenzeller 1990, Uncini et al 1988, Scerbo et al 1992, Kunimoto et al 1992). As argued by Gifford (Gifford 1998, p. 84), the individual undergoing a manual therapy procedure may well be processing the event as a relative 'threat', feel a bit uncertain or uncomfortable, and hence mediate an increase in SNS activation.

Thus an additional proposal for these results is that they may well reflect the variable but possibly powerful psychological impact of the manoeuver in addition to the tissue, segmental and brain stem feedback and feedforward mechanisms that the authors suggest. The point is that the activity of the dedicated brain stem sympathetic compartments and those relating to nociceptor modulation are powerfully influenced by higher centres. The way we perceive the situation we are in and the sensory information we 'receive' is a primary driver of these systems' activity.

In the studies cited that investigate the effects of various techniques on the SNS activity, what needs to be appreciated is the physical differences between the 'treatment' condition, the 'placebo' condition, and the 'control' conditions. The treatment condition involves the well controlled application of the technique under investigation; the 'placebo' condition involves the exact same physical interaction as the treatment condition (physical touch, as well as interaction and communication) except that the actual movement of the technique is not done. In other words, the therapist applies their hands to the patient for the same amount of time as the technique takes, but does not push and let go to produce the treatment oscillation effect. The 'control' condition involves putting the patient in the same position as the treatment condition and the placebo condition, but no hands are applied (for example, see Vincenzino et al 1996). The difficulties of producing a 'placebo' and 'control' group for this type of research are acknowledged. However, to an observer with a bias towards a psychological interpretation, what appears to be being analysed is the psychological impact of three very novel and odd situations. The psychological impact is being reflected in the activity and outward response of the SNS. One would imagine that all three conditions are open to quite varied individual responses that would be determined by such things as feeling awkward, feeling psychologically or physically uncomfortable, or feelings of threat or pleasure. Thus one person might feel far more uncomfortable being left alone in the long sit slump (sympathetic slump) position for the control condition than they might in the placebo condition where they are being held. A quite opposite reaction might occur in another individual who perhaps is not comfortable with the person who is touching and moving them. Different reactions might also be expected relating to the subjects previous experiences, too. For example, if some of the subjects were physiotherapists they might feel comfortable with being physically undressed and handled, whereas others might find the situation distressing.

Another consideration is that in all of the slump investigations the contact with the trunk by the operator was on the opposite side of the body to the sympathetic chain being 'tensioned' and focused on. It is known that manual contact on one side of the body tends to increase the sudomotor activity on the contralateral side and inhibit it on the ipsilateral side in normal subjects (Appenzeller 1990). This offers a further level of complexity to interpreting the results of these procedures.

Caution is indicated when accepting results from studies that use skin conductance as a measure of sympathetic activity as they are known to be fraught with technical difficulties and inaccuracies. For example, the responses are known to habituate as well as being influenced by many factors that are independent of the SNS (Uncini et al 1988, Scerbo et al 1992, Kunimoto et al 1992, Janig 1993, Mathias & Bannister 1993). Mathias and Bannister (1993) have even gone so far as to suggest that for these reasons it is unsuitable to use these measures in clinical trials.

The other measurement recorded throughout the experiments was temperature change, used by the researchers as an indicator of alterations in vasomotor activity. Variable responses were noted in all the studies under scrutiny, with only one showing significant reductions indicating vasoconstriction (see Chiu & Wright 1996, Peterson et al 1993). The results seem to be at variance with the overview of the work provided by Vincenzino and Wright (2002). Here, the authors claim that substantial increases in cutaneous vasomotor activity occur. There appears to be a degree of ambiguity with the interpretation of the results and readers are urged to consult the individual studies cited.

Even so, the validity of this measurement has been questioned. For example, Janig (1993) stated that in experimental conditions, 'the skin temperature is not necessarily correlated with the activity in sympathetic vasoconstrictor neurons. This most probably also applies to equivalent clinical situations but is generally ignored.' He concludes with the important clinical caveat that, 'it is not correct to conclude on the basis of the cold feet or hands of patients that there is a high sympathetic tone or hypersympathetic activity.'

It is important to note that in all the studies the temperature monitoring probe was placed on the dorsum of the hand, a position which is likely to produce confounding results due to the well established fact that the dorsum of the hand has both an active vasodilation and vasoconstriction system under the direct control of the SNS (Bell 1983, Lindblad et al 1990, Johnson 1995). Simply swapping the recording probes around so that conductance was measured posteriorly and temperature anteriorly may have improved the validity of the tests but would still be fraught with confounding variables. Slater (2001) recently indicated caution when making interpretations about sympathetic functioning from these or similar studies.

Vicenzino and Wright (see Vincenzino et al 1998 & 1999) have investigated and proposed a hypothesis to explain the pain relieving effects of mobilisation techniques used in manual therapy. They have used data from their many studies to suggest that the apparent sympathetic excitation noted may be linked with an increase in activity of the dorsal portion of the periaqueductal grey matter in the midbrain with consequent descending inhibition of the spinal cord. They suggest that this involves the non-opioid predominantly noradrenergic lateral column pathways (reviewed by Wright 2002). Whilst a feasible and important suggestion it remains an untested theory and in view of the above criticisms may be based in part on work over which there has to remain a few questions. What is certain is that any single modality is unlikely to exert its analgesic effects via a single line labeled specific pathway such as this (personal communication, P. D. Wall , London, 2001.) What has begun is excellent, but clearly more work is needed to further clarify the situation.

Discussion 2: Models of care—plea for an ordered approach

The most striking observation from this review of the literature is the lack of depth and breadth. There is a lot of work that needs to be done and the hole left by the lack of controlled clinical trials is significantly large to leave little in the way of informed guidance.

CRPS, as its name suggests, is indeed complex and multifactorial. Little wonder that most of us feel a sense of dread and even inadequacy when faced by patients with such extreme sensitivity and disability. Pleasingly, the CRPS Guidelines for Therapy, Consensus Report written by Stanton-Hicks and colleagues (1998) offers a way forward and we re-iterate an earlier suggestion that it is essential reading (see Fig. 5.1.) There are several key points worth highlighting:

- The report summarises current thinking and the consensus position of the International Association for the Study of Pain. It offers clear diagnostic criteria and explains many of the common symptoms of the condition as well as therapy guidance.
- The report provides a multidisciplinary algorithm for management with a central physical therapy based core whose primary goal is reactivation and return of function (see Chapters 6 & 7.)
- Supported on either side of this central core of physical therapy/ reactivation is a requirement for appropriately timed 'medical' and 'psychological' interventions.
- A stepped approach to management that is time dependent is viewed as essential.

The medical interventions listed include the use of:

- *Medications* early on i.e. NSAIDS, opioids, tricyclic antidepressants, alpha-2 agonists, sodium ion channel blocking agents. If these prove inadequate or there is no response the algorithm moves on to:
- '*Blocking procedures*' (+/- medications), listed as: focal, sympathetic, regional, epidural, and pumps. The last tier of intervention then shifts to:

- *'Neurostimulation'* (+/- medications), being either peripheral or epidural.

The supporting psychological interventions proposed include: *Counselling* that deals with expectations, motivation, control, family and 'diary'; *Behaviour*; *Relaxation*; *Imagery*; *Hypnosis*; and *Coping Skills*.

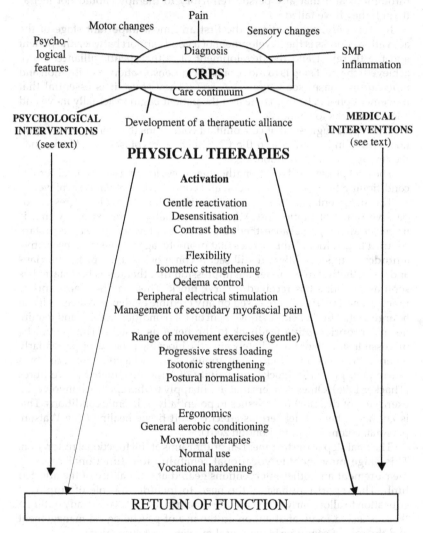

Fig. 5.1 A slightly modified version of the algorithm of management suggested by Stanton-Hicks et al 1998.

Adapted from: Stanton-Hicks et al 1998 Complex regional pain syndromes: guidelines for therapy. The Clinical Journal of Pain 14:155–166.

The authors suggest that 'failure' to achieve improvement after three weeks of the commencement of each stage (see Fig. 5.1) indicates the need for involvement of these other specialties in the management process. Importantly, they point out that patients require maximum support throughout and that any person refractory to therapy should not feel as though they have failed.

Interestingly, they indicate the first and most important stage of the activation process is the development of a good rapport between the patient and the therapist and the development of a 'therapeutic alliance.' Once achieved, the next step is to move onto the desensitisation, mobilisation and motivation phase (see Chapters 6 & 7.) They state 'it is essential that movement phobia be overcome and the patient begin to actually move and allow the limbs to be touched.'

The report suggests that concomitant conditions that continue to 'input' nociceptive information into the CNS such as myofascial problems, may require appropriate attention.

The next phase involves strengthening, stress loading and general aerobic conditioning to support the general and continued reactivation achieved.

The statement that 'It is particularly important to avoid aggressive or passive range of motion (ROM) tests, especially in an extremity that is insensate after regional anaesthetic blockade' is noteworthy since it is in stark contrast to traditional approaches that promote 'aggressive' and insensitive attitudes to this condition. It still seems common for therapists, clinicians and anaesthetists to be under the impression that therapy is best started as soon as someone has received a nerve block. This may be inappropriate practice and is certainly not based on any credible evidence available. It can be argued that the benefits of movement on this condition involve and require normal proprioceptive feedback to the nervous system. This would be impossible during or immediately after the blocking procedure, particularly where there has been a tourniquet applied since ischaemia, produced by a tourniquet, primarily blocks the activity of large myelinated nerve fibres (Thacker 1996). Other dangers that might apply to this approach involve the exercising of dysfunctional tissues in potentially ischaemic conditions. This is known to have a deleterious effect on soft tissue healing (Tim Watson, personal communication, London 2001).

The final step of the treatment algorithm aims at full functional restoration. This stage may include vocational rehabilitation, functional capacity measurement and other interventions geared at normal use of the affected limb. The report emphasises the need to include the role of employee education to allow early, albeit modified, return to work. As already outlined there is also a focus of attention on the use of psychological management and the role of cognitive behavioural management strategies.

The authors state clearly that the biggest obstacle to patient progression is pain and subsequent fear avoidance (see Part 2 in Volume 1 of this series.) They make a clear statement that unacceptable pain requires effective treatment and this is a key indicator for the need for pharmocotherapy, regional blocks, neurostimulation etc. Thus, while physical function is the driver for the algorithm, interventions beyond those outlined in Figure 5.1 are only implemented to allow continued progression. The report is important and unique in that it sets out a broad based multidisciplinary rationale for appropriate treatment selection and progression.

The report usefully outlines in moderate detail the pharmacological and invasive procedures listed above. It also gives some evidence for and against their use and their known efficacy. Mechanisms of action and dosage are briefly outlined and a 'quick guide' is provided to this massive topic. Special attention is given to the topic of CRPS in children, not only with respect to direct management but also to the support and involvement of parents. Specific references are included offering a good first stop for the interested reader.

The recommendations of this report are as yet unproven. However, it is an exciting piece of work for physiotherapists whose input forms the central core of the reactivation process. It is also a rational, well structured and staged approach. In so doing, it takes physiotherapy away from the haphazard trial and error approaches discussed earlier and for which we seem best known. An excellent start for physiotherapy would be to implement the approach and, at some stage, audit and publish outcomes. If proven to be of value it would serve to challenge trends towards unstructured multi-interventions. Here of course, outcomes are impossible to ascribe accurately to one aspect, one intervention or one modality that might be involved in the care. The advice here is to not be charmed by those who advocate easily achieved outcomes using single modalities as core components of their approaches (see Muramatsu et al 1998, as a typical example). Rather, see CRPS, defined by its very nature, as a complex and multifactorial problem that requires a multifactorial, open minded and compassionate approach.

Conclusion

Three main issues arise with CRPS:

1. Proof of the efficacy of physiotherapy modalities and skills in treatment and management is clearly lacking.
2. Until relatively recently, there has not been a clear framework on which to base any intervention. Whether a particular modality works, whatever the discipline, may be largely down to hope, faith, and luck. Patients with CRPS and many patients with other chronic pains, if medicine is honest, are dumped onto physiotherapy. We are the option that takes a bit of time up and moves the difficult patient out of the consulting room hopefully never to return. The proposals of Stanton-Hicks et al (1998) that were reviewed above provide a constructive, multidisciplinary and multidimensional approach that is bathed in strong mutual cross-disciplinary respect. The hope is that all those involved will be interested in playing a part in patient outcomes and as a result work together for

this common goal. The guidelines are clear, graded, and have long term objectives that seem sound and exciting and are a logical option to adopt. What is pleasing is that the right sort of physiotherapy provides the core component of therapy.

3. If the approach proposed by Stanton-Hicks et al (1998) is agreed and adopted it means that mechanistic, tissue targeted and modality dominated therapies, that are the mainstay of most current physiotherapy treatments, and still form a dominant part of training, will have to take a significant back seat in the future management of patients with conditions like CRPS. There are a great many new skills to learn, but most challenging of all is the appreciation and application of important new models of care (see Chapter 8 this volume and Muncey chapters in Volumes 4 and 2).

REFERENCES

Appenzeller O 1990 The Autonomic Nervous System. An Introduction to the Basic and Clinical Concepts, 4th edn. Elsevier, Amsterdam

Bell C 1983 Vasodilator neurons supplying skin and skeletal muscle of the limbs. Journal of the Autonomic Nervous System 7:257–262

Boas R 1999 Workshop Presentation, 9th World Congress on Pain. International Association for the Study of Pain. Austria

Carlson LR, Watson HK 1988 Treatment of reflex sympathetic dystrophy using the stress loading program. Journal of Hand Therapy 1:149–154

Chan CS, Chow SP 1981 Electroacupuncture in the treatment of post-traumatic dystrophy (Sudeck's atrophy). British Journal of Anaesthesia 53:899–902

Charlton JE 1991 Managagement of sympathetic pain. In: Wells JCD, Woolf CJ (eds) Pain Mechanisms and Management. British Medical Bulletin 47 (3):601–618

Chiu TW, Wright A 1996 To compare the effects of different rates of application of a cervical mobilisation technique on sympathetic outflow to the upper limb in normal subjects. Manual Therapy 1:4:198–203

Ernst E, Resch L, Fialka V, Ritter-Dittrich D, Alcamioglu Y, Chen O, Leitha T, Kluger R 1995 Traditional acupuncture for reflex sympathetic dystrophy: A randomised sham-controlled, double blind trial. Acupuncture in Medicine 13(2):78–81

Fitzpatrick AF 2000 Clinical Practice Guidelines. Reflex sympathetic dystroph/ complex regional pain syndrome. Reflex Sympathetic Dystrophy Association of America

Frazer FW 1978 Persistent post sympathetic pain treated by connective tissue massage. Physiotherapy 64(7):211–212

Fredorczyk J 1997 The role of physical agents in modulating pain. Journal of Hand Therapy 10:110–121

Gifford LS 1998 Output mechanisms. In: Gifford LS (ed) Topical Issues in Pain 1. Whiplash—science and management. Fear-avoidance beliefs and behaviour. CNS Press, Falmouth 81–91

Grunert BK, Devine CA, Sanger JR, Matloub HS, Green D 1990 Thermal self-regulation for pain control in reflex sympathetic dystrophy syndrome. Journal of Hand Surgery 15A (4):615–618

Hannington-Kiff JG 1984 Pharmacological target blocks in hand surgery and rehabilitation. Journal of Hand Surgery 9B(1):29–36

Harden RN 2000 A clinical approach in complex regional pain syndrome. Clinical Journal of Pain 16:S26–S32

Harding V 1999 The role of movement in acute pain. In: Max M (ed) Pain—an updated review. Refresher course syllabus. IASP Press, Seattle 159–169

Hardy MA, Hardy SGP 1997 Reflex sympathetic dystrophy: The clinicians perspective. Journal of Hand Therapy 10:137–150

Hareau J 1996 What makes treatment for reflex sympathetic dystrophy successful? Journal of Hand Therapy 9:367–370

Harris W, Wagnon RJ 1987 The effects of chiropractic adjustments on distal skin temperature. Journal of Manipulative and Physiological Therapeutics 12 (2):57–60

Headley B 1987 Historical perspective of causalgia. Management of sympathetically maintained pain. Physical Therapy 67 (9):1370–1374

Hooshmand H 1993 Chronic pain: Reflex sympathetic dystrophy prevention and management. CRC Press. Boca Raton

Janig W 1993 Pain and the autonomic nervous system: Pathophysiological mechanisms. In: Bannister R, Mathias C J (eds) Autonomic Failure, 3rd edn. Oxford University Press, Oxford

Johnson JM, Pergola PE, Liao FK, Kellog DL, Crandall CG 1995 Skin of the dorsal aspect of the human hands and fingers possess an active vasodilator system. American Journal of Physiology 267:948–954

Kappler RE, Kelso AF 1984 Thermographic studies of skin temperature in patients receiving osteopathic manipulation treatment for peripheral nerve problems. Journal of the American Osteopathic Association 84 (1):126–127

Kunimoto M, Kirno K, Karlson T, Wallin BG 1992 Non linearity of skin resistance to intraneural electrical stimulation of sudomotor nerves. Acta Physiologie Scandinavia 146 (3):385–392

Lampen-Smith RA 1997 Complex regional pain syndrome I (RSD) and the physiotherapeutic intervention. New Zealand Journal of Physiotherapy 4:19–23

Larson NL, Watson MW, Kelso AF 1980 Effectiveness of manipulative treatments for parasthesias with peripheral nerve involvement. Journal of the American Osteopathic Association 80 (3):114(Abs)

Leo KC 1983 Use of electrical stimulation at acupuncture points for the treatment of reflex sympathetic dystrophy in a child. Physical Therapy 63:957–959

Lindblad LE, Ekenvall L, Klingstedt C 1990 Neural regulation of vascular tone and cold induced vasoconstriction in the human finger skin. Journal of the Autonomic Nervous System 30:169–174

Low A, Reed A 1994 Electrotherapy Explained: Principles and practice 2nd edn. Butterworth-Hienemann, Oxford

Low J 1994 Electrotherapeutic modalities. In: Wells PE, Frampton V, Bowsher D (eds) Pain Management by Physiotherapy. Butterworth Heinemann, Oxford 140–176

Main CJ, Spanswick CC 2000 Pain Management. An interdisciplinary approach. Churchill Livingstone, Edinburgh

Martin D (1996) Interferential therapy. In: Kitchen S, Bazin S (eds) Clayton's Electrotherapy 10th edn. Saunders, London

Mathias CJ, Bannister R 1993 Investigation of autonomic disorders. In : Bannister R, Mathias CJ (eds) Autonomic Failure 3rd edn. Oxford University Press, Oxford

Melzack R 1994 Folk medicine and the sensory modulation of pain. In: Wall PD, Melzack R (eds) Textbook of Pain 3rd edn. Churchill Livingstone, Edinburgh

Muramatsu K, Kawai S, Akino T, Sunago K, Doi K 1998 Treatment of chronic regional pain syndrome using manipulation therapy. Regional Anaesthesia 44(1):189–192

Peterson N, Vincenzino W, Wright A 1993 The effects of a cervical mobilisation technique on sympathetic outflow to the upper limb in normal subjects. Physiotherapy Theory and Practice 9:149–156

Portwood MM, Lieberman JS, Taylor R 1987 Ultrasound treatment of reflex sympathetic dystrophy. Archives of Physical Medicine and Rehabilitation 68:116–118

Savage B 1984 Interferential Therapy. Faber and Faber, London

Scerbo AS, Freedman LW, Raine A, Dawson ME, Venables PH 1992 A major effect of recording site on measurement of electrodermal activity. Psychophysiology 29(2):241–246

Slater H 1991 Adverse neural tension in the sympathetic trunk and sympathetic maintained pain syndromes. In. Proceedings of the Seventh Biennial Conference of the Manipulative Physiotherapist Association of Australia

Slater H 1995 An investigation of the physiological effects of the sympathetic slump on peripheral sympathetic nervous system function in patients with frozen shoulder. In: Shacklock M (ed) Moving in on pain. Butterworth Heinemann, Sydney

Slater H 2001 Vegetatives nervensystem In: Van den Berg F (ed) Angewandte Physiologie: 3 Therapie, Training, Tests. Georg Thieme Verlag, Stuttgart

Slater H, Vincenzino G, Wright A 1994 'Sympathetic slump': The effects of a novel manual therapy technique on peripheral sympathetic nervous system dysfunction. The Journal of Manual and Manipulative Therapy 2 (4):156–162

Slater H, Wright A, Vincenzino G 1993 Physiological effects of the sympathetic slump on peripheral sympathetic nervous system function. In: Integrating Approaches. Proceedings of the Eighth Biennial Conference of the Manipulative Physiotherapist Association of Australia

Stanton-Hicks M 1998 Management of patients with complex regional pain syndromes. PSNS SIG Newsletter. IASP Press, Seattle

Stanton-Hicks M, Baron R, Boas R, Gordh T, Harden RN, Hendler N, Koltzenberg M, Raj P, Wilder R 1998 Complex regional pain syndrome: Guidelines for therapy. Clinical Journal of Pain 14:155–166

Stanton-Hicks M, Janig W, Hassenbusch S, Haddox J D, Boas R, Wilson P 1995 Reflex sympathetic dystrophy: Changing concepts and taxonomy. Pain 63:127–133

Taylor-Mullins PA 1989 Management of common chronic pain problems of the hand. Physical Therapy. 69 (12):1050–1058

Thacker MA 1995 The effect of 'self sympathetic slumping' on peripheral sympathetic nervous system activity. MSc Thesis. University College London. London University

Thacker MA 1996 Early intervention in the management of complex regional pain syndrome I. Does it make a difference? Abstract, Pain Society of Great Britain Annual Scientific Meeting

Thomas D 1996 Physiotherapy and rehabilitation of upper extremity reflex sympathetic dystrophy. Clinical Orthopaedics 1 (2):339–360

Uncini A, Pulman SL, Lovelace RE, Gambi D 1988 The sympathetic skin response: Normal values, elucidation of afferent components and application limits. Journal of Neurological Science 87 (2-3):299–306

Vincenzino B, Collins D, Wright A 1996 The initial effects of a cervical spine manipulative physiotherapy treatment on the pain and dysfunction of lateral epicondylalgia. Pain 68: 69–74

Vincenzino G, Cartwright T, Collins DM, Wright A 1999 An investigation of stress and pain perception during manual therapy in asymptomatic subjects. European Pain Journal 3:13–18

Vincenzino G, Collins D, Wright A 1994 Sudomotor changes influenced by neural mobilisation techniques in asymptomatic subjects. The Journal of Manual and Manipulative Therapy 2(2):66–74

Vincenzino G, Collins DM, Benson HAE, Wright A 1998 The interrelationship between manipulation induced analgesia and sympathoexcitation. Journal of Manipulative and Physiological Therapeutics 7(12): 448–453

Vlaeyen JWS, Linton S J 2000 Fear-avoidance and its consequences in chronic musculoskeletal pain: A state of the art. Pain 85(3):317–332

Walker SM, Cousins MJ 1996 Complex regional pain syndromes: Including 'Reflex sympathetic dystrophy' and 'Causalgia'. Anaesthesia and Intensive Care 25:113–125

Watson HK, Carlson LR 1987 Treatment of RSD of the hand with an 'active stress-loading' program. Journal of Hand Surgery 12A:779–785

Withrington RH, Wynn Parry CB 1984 The management of painful peripheral nerve disorders. Journal of Hand Surgery. 9B (12):24–28

Wright A 2002 Neurophysiology of pain and pain modulation. In: Strong J, Unruh A, Wright A et al (eds) Pain: A textbook for therapists. Churchill Livingstone, Edinburgh 43–64

Zusman M 1995 Sympathetic responses to passive movement manoeuvres. Proceedings of the Ninth Biennial Conference of the Manipulative Physiotherapists Association of Australia

Assessment and case management of complex regional pain syndrome

SUZANNE BROOK

Introduction

In the UK health service there exists a great contrast between medical and self management approaches to musculoskeletal pain problems. A medical approach does not place importance on the individual's experiences, beliefs and thoughts. In this chapter I will use a case history to discuss my work with chronic, complex regional pain syndrome (CRPS). The case utilises a self management perspective, illustrating the role of the individuals thoughts, fears and beliefs concerning their pain and their future.

Presentation

I first met Brian whilst he was an inpatient at a specialist hospital in London, having been admitted for further investigations into his chronic pain. I received the referral following a case conference between a neurologist and his team and a pain consultant. Their conclusion was that an assessment by a specialist pain management physiotherapist would be valuable.

It is unusual for me to see inpatients, partly as time does not allow for it but, more importantly, because admission for medical management of chronic pain problems conflicts with the approach used within pain management departments. It places the patient in a difficult position between pain investigation and pain alleviation (medical model) and, conversely, pain management (self-management model). Normally I would have suggested that an outpatient appointment after discharge would be more beneficial for Brian. However, Brain was told that he would be seen by the 'pain team' before he left so I felt it would be unfair on him to change it. The inpatient assessment was made as a one-off but it was made clear to all concerned that further management, if appropriate, would be on an outpatient basis.

Discussing the situation with the medical team prior to my assessment, it became apparent that it was their frustration at being unable to do anything for Brain that led them to ask for my assessment. I could not help feeling frustrated at their perception of the pain management approach. I had effectively been presented to Brian 'as the last hope' and not even given the opportunity to suggest when his appointment for assessment would be most beneficial. This is one example that highlights the limited understanding of a pain management/self management approach for chronic pain.

The referral

The referral I received stated that Brian had had a knee injury two years previously. His knee had been placed in a full leg Plaster of Paris cast for four months; it was removed for a month and then re-plastered for another three months, during which period Brian was diagnosed with complex regional pain syndrome to the left lower limb (see Chapter 2 for discussion on immobility).

The current admission was for 'observation' (of what I am not sure) and to carry out further diagnostic tests. The tests included four nerve conduction studies that were designated 'normal'. Bone density studies showed reduced levels in the lumbar spine, left hip, tibial plateau, distal extremities of the fibula and tibia and the tarsus. Bone scans showed a reduced vascularity in the left lower limb.

There was no mention of how Brian was coping with his pain, any effects that it had on his mood, how he felt about being admitted to the hospital to be observed and tested, or what his expectations were of his stay and for his future.

Brian was described as a young lad whose case was 'interesting but nothing is really wrong except severe muscle weakness, a bit of pain but a lot of fear.' Bone density loss was acknowledged but attributed to the absence of weight bearing (but this would not be the cause of the pain.) The suggestion from the medical team was that there was no organic reason to explain Brian's pain.

This type of opinion can often lead to bias during the assessment process. Since no reasonable organic pathology was found the belief held by the medical and nursing team on the wards was to covertly label Brian as a malingerer, with the implication that his pain was not real. The complexity of chronic pain was apparently not understood. Unfortunately, once the reality of someone's pain is under question, those assessing and managing the patient treat them differently, behave differently, perhaps not taking them seriously, nor fully listening to them or becoming dismissive of what they say and do. This may happen unconsciously and is a response to a belief whose basis is rarely challenged. Brian had no doubt become aware of the negative way he was being thought of on the ward. In this sort of situation patients who feel that their veracity is being challenged often tend to increase the very behaviour that the carers associate with 'unreal' pain, which further reinforces their beliefs.

In order not to perpetuate Brian's feeling of not being believed, a careful assessment approach was required. It also needed to be acknowledged that some of his behaviour would be more linked to his mood, his understandable upset about what was happening, his worries about his admission, and his fear of movement and activity. For these reasons I suggested that a joint assessment by the pain physiotherapist and a pain psychologist would be most beneficial. The suggestion that a clinical psychologist needed to be involved had to be made carefully to the neurology team on the ward as it was important to avoid reinforcing the idea that the patient was deliberately exaggerating his problems or that we considered them psychogenic. The suggestion was therefore made that, bearing in mind the effects on the patient of previous poor treatment and management outcomes, it would be helpful for Brian to have the opportunity to meet a psychologist who could then assess the impact the pain had had on his lifestyle and that this might lead to utilising strategies that would improve his mood, coping, and functioning. The inclusion of a psychologist is in sharp contrast to a psychiatrist whose skills may be utilised in the assessment and medical management of psychological diseases and disorders. Psychiatrists are often asked by medical teams to determine whether patients have real pain; this is not the role of psychologists.

Medical history

The medical notes gave a clear history of a 19 year old male, who had a soft tissue injury to his left knee whilst attending college. He had visited his local casualty department two days later to seek pain relief and for reassurance that there was no serious injury. X-rays revealed no bony injury. Brian was diagnosed as having a soft tissue injury and referred to the local orthopaedic clinic. At this clinic he was placed in a below knee plaster cast. When the plaster was removed four months later there was no change in pain report. Then, following some treatment at the local pain clinic, Brain's leg was re-plastered for a further three months. According to the medical notes it was at this point that Brian was diagnosed as having complex regional pain syndrome to the left lower limb. Upon removal of the plaster eight months after the initial injury, Brian was referred to his local physiotherapy department. A comment in the notes said: 'Treatment was unsuccessful due to the patient's poor compliance.' One month later Brian's GP referred him to both an orthopaedic surgeon and a neurologist at a specialist hospital in London, at which point I was asked to assess Brian.

Physiotherapy assessment

Whilst visiting the ward to see Brian's notes I noticed that he spent all his time lying on his bed with his left leg over two pillows. The nurses commented on their frustration with his apparent laziness and contentment at having things done for him. This reinforced my initial preference to meet Brian outside the ward environment, to remove any suggestions or feelings on his side that I colluded with the medical staff. It was difficult not to form a negative mental picture of him, his behaviour, and his presentation from what I had been told about him by the doctors, nurses and other physiotherapists working on the ward. I needed to provide a different format of assessment, a different approach and environment.

It was very important for me to avoid making inflexible assumptions. While this can often be difficult to do with many patients, prior assumptions are an important barrier to helping since rigid pre-conceived thoughts and interpretations may mislead the assessment and limit one's ability to gain better insight into the patient's thoughts and hopes about their future.

From the brief I was given, my expectations were to find a young man on a ward in an intimidating environment. He would probably be aware that he was presenting a challenge to the staff and might even feel scared and confused. This is not so much a criticism of the staff, but more a criticism of the consequences of the medical approach.

Appreciating what a patient might have been told or advised to do and the possible consequences for them is worthwhile. Brian was likely to have received many conflicting messages with regard to immobilisation, exercise, and fitness. Immobilisation for such a long period could only have reinforced the idea that his leg should not be moved. His current admission would possibly have acted to increase his fears about the severity and rarity of his condition. It would also be realistic to expect Brian to be unsure of my role, bearing in mind not just his previous history concerning immobilisation, but the unplanned nature of our meeting. I had no specific information on what his previous physiotherapy had involved except that 'it had not been successful.' This may only be the patient's perception, but an awareness of his previous experience with physiotherapy was important, if only so I could differentiate my approach from previous therapies, which are likely to have been more modality based, pain relief focused, passive, and hence 'medical' approaches.

It was agreed that Brian would visit my office in the pain management department. This gave us the opportunity to meet Brian in a setting away from the ward where it would be easier to introduce a different approach to helping Brian understand and manage his pain more successfully.

The role that the psychologist would take throughout the assessment was discussed prior to meeting Brian. Bearing in mind Brain's age and the obvious implications that the presence of a psychologist might have, it was decided that I would lead the assessment and the psychologist would be present to ask occasional loose and open questions, as appropriate. Although the presence of the psychologist could be confusing at first, we felt that it would help to move the discussion towards the impact and effects that the pain was having. For example it is often helpful in these early stages of a self management approach to acknowledge with the patient that having pain for such a long time normally affects people's confidence, and their moods and hopes for the future.

Brian hopped in using two crutches, with his left knee held at 90° flexion, weight bearing through his right leg only. Understandably he looked unsure and nervous. Brian sat mainly weight-bearing on his right side, rotated his upper body to the right, and held his left foot off the floor with the back of his left knee held away from the edge of the seat.

After we had introduced ourselves, I explained why we were both meeting with him and why it was occurring in the pain management department. As Brian had not expected to meet either of us during his admission I explained why it had been decided to arrange the assessment, and why the psychologist was present. The psychologist went on to state that it was not because the doctors did not know what to do (it would not be helpful for Brian to sense further their feelings of despair), nor that we felt that he was making his pain up or exaggerating it. The main thing was to assess the possible benefits of a different approach. The overall aim of our introduction was for Brian to feel that we were different, that our approach would be different from those of both the medical team and the previous physiotherapist, and that a different approach needed to be portrayed through the questions asked and the reactions given to his answers. Hopefully our reactions would be seen as showing more understanding and empathy than any he had previously received.

I was unsure of the ordering of my questions and chose to ask about his pain history early on. On other occasions I ask about this later and enquire about previous physiotherapy and current perceptions about exercise and movement first. Regardless of the exact order of the questions, the psychologist and I needed to let Brian tell us about his experiences early in the assessment. In this way we could use his language from the outset and via this allow him to feel that we understood what had happened and what he was going through.

I asked Brian how he was finding his stay in hospital. He was hesitant in replying and looked miserable, saying, 'I'm bored. I can't understand why they have brought me in for so long, surely I could have had all these tests done in a day.' Brian did not comment on the results of the tests or his feeling about having them done, but rather on why he had to be away from home. This illustrated Brian's low confidence, but which was seen by the medical team as his passivity. Brian's low level of confidence remained apparent throughout our meeting. His trust in the doctors had previously been unquestioned and I sensed a feeling of frustration and confusion at their inability to alleviate his pain. When I asked if that was how he felt, Brian repeated that he was bored, that he was missing his family, and hospital food was awful. (This highlighted why patients are not usually seen during an inpatient stay. To remove someone from their home environment for medical investigations may be important but is unhelpful if one's aim is to help the patient to be more involved in managing their condition.)

It became apparent very quickly that Brian felt like an experiment: things were being done without his understanding (and arguably without his full involvement.) Yet Brian previously had not questioned any of his treatment, in fact he had asked for further plastering to occur (this had not been apparent from the medical notes.) This of course was not his fault; it simply reflected an understandable lay belief concerning pain and its management. His total trust in and compliance with medical care could be judged as passivity (unfairly in my view), but the responses of those in the medical team who possess more factually based beliefs can also be questioned. Further discussion of previous medical treatment is not the aim of this chapter, but what is clear is that any future explanations given to Brian needed to address why his treatments did not cure him, why all the tests had not lead to the alleviation of his pain, and the role and importance of self-management. What became clear was that all through Brian's treatment the possibility of his effective role in his own management and the perception that he could manage things himself with advice and encouragement were greatly doubted. Strategies he may have found useful had not been explored or reinforced and at no time was Brian given the impression he could take responsibility for his pain and health.

During our meeting Brian presented as very despondent ('lazy' as the nurses saw him) but, in the context of how confused he was concerning his admission and previous treatment, his behaviour was hardly surprising. It is invariably more useful to question the label of 'laziness' and redefine it more helpfully as consequence of 'uncertainty.' This illustrates why little value could be placed on descriptions of Brian's behaviour and attitude by the medical staff. His pain needed to be understood in the context of the inter-relationships of the pain, his beliefs and the influence of his environment.

When Brian was asked what he had expected from his stay in hospital he commented that it was for the doctors to do more tests, one for muscles and the other for nerves. He seemed unsure of what the results would imply and the effects they would have upon the treatment or management of his pain. Brian said that he thought they did the tests because they knew what was wrong and then 'surely they could correct it with the right treatment…Now that they have told me nothing is wrong with my nerves they have said I can go home after seeing you.' When we asked Brian how he felt about that, he just shrugged his shoulders. The confusion that this presents is obvious. The admission had suggested to Brian that there would be an explanation and treatment for his pain problem. Being told that there was nothing wrong left him feeling let down, confused and despondent. Again his passivity was seen, but he then went on to question his future: 'This seems like a dead end. What's next, will I be like this for ever?' This was the first time he questioned his management. When both the psychologist and I acknowledged how confusing and frightening that must be, he nodded. He appeared disillusioned about his future and unsure of how he could go forward when he had obvious leg wasting and pain, but yet no understanding of his pain and why it persisted.

Despite my initial aim to ask Brian about his pain onset first, his comments about his future and concerns about his pain led me to ask him about what he thought was wrong, what was causing the pain. 'Bearing in mind all the doctors you have seen and the things said, and with your own ideas, what do you think happened to your leg and what's causing the pain to carry on?' He replied slowly and with some uncertainty, 'They talked about muscle weakness because I have not used the leg much, also that the blood and nerves may be wrong—but yet the tests say the opposite, I find it all confusing.' 'And do you have any ideas for why the pain has lasted?' Brian sighed and, whilst looking down, said, 'They say its because I didn't use it enough at the beginning and therefore the muscles stopped working—but why did they put it in plaster? [his tone was rising] They are the doctors, not me.' The question Brain raised needed to be acknowledged, even if it could not be answered. One needs to be careful not to disagree openly with previous treatment (even when you do disagree), but statements such as, 'They did what they thought was the right thing to do at the time' and 'Ideas have changed a great deal since then' can provide the opportunity to discuss more helpful and current thoughts concerning management.

In order to allow Brian to give as much information as he wanted he was asked open-ended questions, but it was obviously difficult for him and he gave short answers with little elaboration. This could have been for several reasons. One may have been his uncertainty as to how his answers would be perceived, particularly when previous experiences he had had with clinicians might have left him feeling that he should not ask questions or challenge the decisions made. Here, Brain was a 19 year old who was with two older females whom he had known for only a short while; most young adults would surely respond the same way. Rapport and trust would take time to build up.

I went on to ask Brain about what had happened initially and what had happened since. I explained, 'The reason I ask this is that, although I have read your notes, it is much more helpful for me to hear how *you* saw it rather than the doctors, as I am interested in slightly different things, especially your thoughts concerning treatment and your future. As a physiotherapist I am also interested in hearing about what you do now and what you did do physically.' He was slow to answer, possibly unsure of why I was asking something so many others had not asked. He explained that he was in the first year of agricultural college at the time and had been moving some equipment when he hit his knee. I asked what he thought had happened to his leg at the time. He thought he had really damaged something, so returned home and took the rest of the day off. Later, he saw his GP who gave him anti-inflammatories and advised rest.

I asked Brian if anyone had asked him for his own opinion on what had happened and what he thought was wrong. He seemed surprised by the question and said no, he didn't really understand what had happened, 'I don't know, possibly the muscles have stopped working and the nerves are stuck to them. The pain gets worse if I move it so I don't do much. The doctors said all the tests were normal and it was no surprise that my bones were weak, so I am not sure what is wrong or what that meant.' Brian then said that he 'had felt very trusting in doctors but I am not sure now.' When I enquired why that was, he talked of his uncertainty about the length of time he had been in the plaster cast. At the time he had just wanted pain relief but with hindsight felt it may have made his pain worse. This showed insight on his part but I did not feel it appropriate to agree strongly with the comment, as I was yet to understand how that made him feel. I then asked Brian to go back a bit and tell me about what happened concerning the decision to put him in plaster. The question was asked with care as I did not want to imply that he might be to blame for not using the leg enough after the injury—it was already clear that he had been blamed by the doctors for his ongoing pain.

With further prompting he explained that the pain increased over the two days after the injury. He felt his foot became 'stuck in a straight line' (plantar flexion). Two days later his parents took him to casualty, where he was X-rayed. Brian was given the diagnosis of a soft tissue injury to the left knee, given a referral for the orthopaedic clinic in 10 days' time, and told to rest. Unfortunately the advice from two doctors to rest and the pending referral to an orthopaedic department reinforced the idea that something was seriously wrong, despite all physical tests being clear, and a soft tissue injury being diagnosed. It is not surprising that Brian limited his movement completely, rested during the day, and did not return to college.

Asking Brian about his activity level immediately after the injury would allow further insight into his beliefs about pain and movement. He had continued to rest, and then, accompanied by his parents, attended the orthopaedic appointment where he was placed in a full leg plaster (non-weight bearing) for the next four months. He remembered that the pain stayed in his left knee and especially in his left foot. Brian remained off college and rested at home. At the follow-up appointment four months later, the plaster was removed and Brian talked of his surprise at how thin his leg was. The doctors told him that the muscles had wasted away and probably the nerves and blood supply had been damaged in the injury. It was understandable how, without further clarification, Brian came to believe that these changes were a consequence of the initial injury and not the period of immobilisation.

It was at this point that he was diagnosed as having complex regional pain syndrome but it was clear that Brian was unaware of the term, as he had not used it once during the assessment. Upon asking him, he seemed unsure of it but commented that someone here had mentioned something about 'regional pain.' When we brought the conversation back to Brian's time at the orthopaedic clinic he talked of his fear that the pain was still there, saying, 'I just wanted them to take the pain away.' From this appointment Brian was referred to his local pain clinic, were he remembered having some injections (two guanethidine blocks) with no benefit. He then said that the pain was unbearable and he 'begged' the doctors to put the plaster back on. It seems therefore that at Brian's request (in the orthopaedic clinic) the plaster was reapplied for a further three months (this time below knee), and he remained non-weight bearing with two elbow crutches.

Three months later the plaster was removed and Brian was referred to the local physiotherapy department. He remembers the doctors telling him that he needed 'intensive physiotherapy.' I enquired as to how he had found the physiotherapy, what they did, and how had it helped. He just said, 'It

150

made me worse, everything they tried hurt more.' Brian commented that no one could touch the leg, as it was so sore, so the physiotherapist had given him exercises for the hip and knee as he had found it impossible to move his left foot. When I asked if he been able to do any of the exercises at home, he shook his head, 'I tried but it made the pain worse.' Brian remained non-weight bearing and continued to use the crutches. He saw the physiotherapist three times before being told that physiotherapy would not help and was discharged. It was after this that his GP referred Brian to the London Hospital for assessment and subsequent admission.

It is obvious from Brian's account that he had had a very passive role during his treatment, even when encouraged to do home exercises. It is also clear that Brian thought that the pain meant something was wrong and it was to be avoided. It can be seen that, from an early stage, Brian's fear of pain associated with movement was strongly reinforced by the referral to the orthopaedic clinic and further immobilisation. Brian could have been questioned about why he allowed, indeed asked for, further plastering to occur. However, our interview revealed that he was unable to remember anyone discussing with him the longer-term effects of immobilisation or that pain did not necessarily mean something was still wrong. To have pressed him further could be to imply that he was to blame for his present state. For me as a physiotherapist, the understandable myths held by Brian, and the unhelpful reinforcement he had received concerning his pain, needed to be re-addressed with more helpful and realistic information, but in order to do that I needed to learn more from Brian about his thoughts and beliefs concerning physiotherapy, exercise, movement and his previous level of fitness, as well as his thoughts about exercise in the future.

Physical and functional observation and assessment

This happened at the end of the assessment, partly to give Brian the opportunity to get to know me but also to learn about his own thoughts and fears and to keep the focus away from a medical approach. On observing Brian's leg it was clear that his calf muscles were very wasted, with a circumference 28 cm up from his ankle joint of only 25 cm. His ankle was held in plantar flexion. He was unable to weight bear on his left leg. He had no movement at the ankle. The left knee movement was greatly restricted with a loss of 40° of extension. Brian rested his knee on its lateral border at all times (including at night when it rested in 50° of flexion, over pillows). He had pain all over his left leg, his left buttock, across his lower back, in both shoulders radiating down the lateral aspects of his arms to his elbows. Brian had no pain in his right leg, thoracic and cervical spine or his lower arms. He described peculiar sensations and intermittent swelling in his left foot.

Large necrotic areas were present over Brian's ankle and calf, which he did not like looking at. The skin otherwise was dry, broken, and with red patches. He was unable to tolerate touch of any sort to the lower limb and preferred to cover the limb with three crepe bandages and his jeans as he felt that this minimised the possibility of it being knocked.

Upon request Brian was able to elicit a flicker of big toe movement. When I asked Brian when he had last noticed that, he said he hadn't been able to do it for weeks. This provided reinforcement for changes that had occurred since the plaster had been removed; hence a link could be made between increase in movement (however slight) and the absence of the plaster. Brian was asked to complete the standard physical fitness assessment, within a controlled environment, but without his crutches. He was initially hesitant but complied when it was explained that it was not a test and that it can be a very helpful measure of progress. He completed a five minute walk covering 80 metres by hopping and using a wall occasionally for support. He managed six stand-ups in a minute and 12 stairs, both carried out by using his right leg only.

Family influences

Brian lives with his family: mum, dad and two older brothers. Both his parents were working, one brother was attending college, and the other was working. Brian was initially seen without his family, which was his choice, but his parents were asked to join us for the last ten minutes of the assessment. Upon meeting his family it was obvious how anxious they were about Brian's management and the lack of effective pain relief. They were also very anxious that any movement would cause further pain. Brian's mother particularly felt that movement should be avoided. It was clear that the family as a whole believed that something was physically wrong but no longer felt the answer was going to come from surgery, more plastering or admissions. I took the opportunity to help Brian explain to his parents what I had told him about a self-management approach and what physiotherapy involved in that context. I also suggested that a lot of the information I would like to discuss with Brian and his parents would differ from what they may have been told in the past. Interestingly, Brian's mother replied that any information would be better than none. She had a good insight into how much of what they thought was right was based on what they believed, not what they had been told since Brian's accident. Just as it was important to learn about Brian's thoughts concerning his pain, so it was important to learn about his family's beliefs. Since his family was in virtually constant contact with Brian they could help him to make changes and persevere with the things we agreed.

Previous history

Brian had previously enjoyed football, which he played four times a week, and also went running once or twice a week. At the time of our first meeting he was doing upper body exercises, mainly free weight lifting, approximately three to four times a week, but said, 'I avoid using my leg as much as possible.' Brian fearfed moving his left hip, knee and foot, and I needed to understand why he held that fear in the context of what he understood to have happened. He had already mentioned that he had been told that the muscles had wasted and the nerves had become 'stuck.' When asked 'What do you think is happening to cause the pain when you try to move it?', Brian looked unsure and said 'It must be the muscles that are wrong, they are so thin, my ankle is stuck and doesn't move at all.' I needed to learn about what Brian thought had happened at the time of injury, as it was clear that his beliefs had affected his management. 'What do you think actually happened when you knocked your knee?' Brian went on to say that he must have bruised something and hit the bone. 'Do you think that the injury has healed?' 'No, otherwise it wouldn't hurt so much.' Of course we know clinically that the soft tissue injury would have healed within a six to twelve week period, but Brian's belief that it had not gave some understanding as to why he avoided moving it.

An initial assessment is not always the best time to 'correct' information that is held by patients. Initially it needs to be collected and viewed in a larger context of how people try to understand what has happened and how they cope. To suddenly tell patients that what they have believed for so long is wrong is to take away the very strategies they currently use to cope with the pain. That is not to say that the information should not be challenged. Once the therapist understands the condition and the patient's beliefs, the patient can be asked if they want to hear and learn about alternative theories of what has happened and what other strategies can replace those held. 'Would you like to know more about what has happened to your leg and what you can do about it now?' or 'Would you like to have the term complex regional pain syndrome explained to you?' These may seem obvious questions but by asking them, the patient immediately has a chance to opt into the management plan and the approach starts to become more self-managing. By linking this to the patient's own hopes, however unrealistic they may appear, we start to develop goals that can be worked towards.

When I asked Brian these questions he was initially doubtful, responding with, 'What can I do about it now?' I went on to explain about the self-management approach used within our department and how we placed him within the model. He seemed intrigued, especially when I enquired about his future hopes. Brian hoped to walk normally again, to return to agricultural college, and to play football. What often needs to be established is whether an individual feels they can achieve their goals and hopes despite the pain continuing. The question, 'Do you think it is possible to gain fitness and move more even if the pain continues?' can be usefully asked. It is equally valuable to ask whether the patient feels their pain will continue or be cured. Although this can be a difficult question, it needs to be asked to gain a sense of how ready the patient is to accept their situation and then take on board a self-managing approach. Someone who places high hopes in gaining a cure from treatment will find a self-management approach very challenging. On the other hand, despite their initial wish to be pain free, someone who has come to realise that a cure is not likely will usually take on board a self-management approach more readily and with more awareness and more realistic expectations.

Brian revealed that he thought he would have pain all his life now and that the doctors would not be able to cure it.

The psychologist

Since Brian presented primarily with physical concerns, the psychologist's role in the assessment was relatively minor. In discussions with the psychologist after the assessment, she felt that Brian was not unduly distressed concerning his pain and further support was not necessary. She felt hopeful that, with the support and strategies I could offer, Brian could make changes successfully, although if later it became apparent that Brian would benefit from psychological help then a referral could be made. Unfortunately during the first assessment no psychological measures were taken, and as no further psychology involvement was planned, further measures were not requested. In hindsight this was a mistake as these measures often help by providing reinforcing evidence for any changes made.

Impressions from the subjective assessment

It became clear that throughout all that had happened, Brian had been a passive recipient. He might once have been called the ideal patient! Now he was the ideal patient to benefit from a self-help approach.

Brian needed to be given up-to-date and realistic information concerning the nature of his pain, its management and possible future expectations. For Brian to achieve his long term goals he needed to become more involved, not only for his well-being but also to ensure maintenance of the changes that he could make. Usefully, Brian responded well to encouragement and words of praise. It was hoped that if those at home could reinforce more helpful behaviours like movement and going out more, then the likelihood of Brian making progress would be maximised.

For physiotherapy intervention to be beneficial, patient and physiotherapist need to discuss the type of activities that would be meaningful for that patient to work on. Countryman and Gekas (1980) stated that '... a patient who has adequate information for participation in decisions that personally affect him or her is less likely to be dissatisfied with the outcome of the treatment.' Therefore the aims of physiotherapy management for Brian needed to be based around his goals, which in turn could only be fully explored once he had all the information pertaining to the methods by which change may be possible.

Management

Education and imparting information

Previous medical management had presented Brian with an explicit message that immobilisation was appropriate, though the inconsistency evident in also suggesting that mobilisation was always important obviously left Brian in an confused position.

It would not have been appropriate or helpful to tell Brian that previous treatment had been inappropriate, misguided, or that it may have been largely responsible for his current problems. New information is best presented to replace the existing held beliefs rather than directly challenge them. For example, comments like 'it is not too late for the body to make changes in a more helpful way, despite what has happened in the past' can be very useful.

The medical terminology that Brian would have heard (perhaps without fully understanding it) during his admission may have added to the already confusing picture. Complicated medical words or over-simplified explanations of pain need to be demystified and comprehensive information given in a way appropriate to the patient. Written and verbal information concerning possible causes of the pain, pain behaviour and the wide-ranging strategies that can be used to increase fitness and improve quality of life should be given. Many chapters in this and other volumes in the series provide useful information that can be reformulated and passed on to patients. The level and speed of information giving should be directed by patients themselves. Clearly we must be careful not to underestimate how much patients need and can cope with in terms of detailed explanations of pain and its future management. Patten and Nelson (1996) carried out a preliminary study of patients' perceptions of aspects of their physical therapy experience and asked: 'Should [physiotherapists] give the patients only what they currently know enough to want for themselves, or should we try to educate them to assume more responsibility for their own on-going health monitoring and health care? Surely our role is to provide the latter?' This component of intervention and management cannot be neglected and often needs to be gone through many times. It will form the foundation for patients feeling more in control of their pain and better equipped with strategies to maintain the changes they make.

Brian's family's concerns about his pain, especially their fear that allowing him to move too much would cause further damage and distress, needed to be challenged. At Brian's request, family members were included in sessions, with written information being taken home and read by the whole family. Time had to be made available for them to ask questions. In particular I needed to help Brian to tell his family what he was doing as well as reviewing progress with them to maximise their involvement. By witnessing that Brian could change his daily routine and increase and cope with new levels of activity the family's confidence would increase, hopefully leading to a more reinforcing environment for further changes. In many ways, this adjustment of the family was just as important as Brian's own recognition of his progress. Achieving physical and functional goals is the best reinforcer of change and the best challenge to any previously unhelpful beliefs and fears about damage, pain and treatments.

Functional recovery

Brian had already stated that his long-term aims were to walk without crutches, to return to college, and to play football. In order for these to become achievable Brian needed to break them down into more manageable shorter-term goals. I needed to give information first so that Brian would know how to do this and how to make judgements concerning appropriate starting points. Brian and his family needed to be given information about Brian's complex regional pain syndrome generally, and possibilities for his future. They also needed strategies to help with managing flare-ups and the confidence to continue despite the pain.

In discussions during his second appointment Brian showed he was aware that in order to achieve his long-term goals he needed to work on many things. A list generated included: an increase in his range of movement in his left foot and knee, a reduction in the sensitivity of his lower limb, a decrease in the use of crepe bandages, an improvement in the skin condition over his left lower limb, an improvement in his balance, and confidence in standing and maintenance and increased general fitness (these are discussed in more detail below).

Brian's own planning skills in breaking down large goals into manageable goals needed to be built upon and encouraged: 'As your long term goal is to walk normally, what do you think you need to work on first?' There is no right or wrong answer, but Brian needed encouragement not to set his expectations too high. Walking without his crutch the next day would be unrealistic but toe touching a soft surface would be a good start. For Brian to continue with a problem-solving approach he needed to learn how to make the decisions himself; criticism from me or any attempt to change his goals would only reduce his confidence further. Once Brian had developed the ability to break activities down and problem-solve challenging areas, he would be in a position to need me less. A successful outcome is not necessarily indicated by large functional changes but rather by the patient having a sound grasp of the concepts he will need to go on making the changes.

(Details concerning exercise implementation are discussed in the next chapter.)

Confidence

Brian's low level of self-confidence, evident during assessment, needed to be increased. Successful goal achievement is a fundamental process that gradually challenges fears and increases confidence. It is important for goal attainment to be planned and realised in a systematic, controlled and supported way. Encouraging him to fill in his own exercise sheets and to plan and write his own graded activity sheets further boosted his confidence. It is important that patients learn problem-solving skills and how to plan and execute goal-orientated programmes. The aim is for patients to learn to attribute the changes and goals achieved to themselves, not to the therapist. This is an important key to successful self management, maintenance of progress and prevention of repeated phone calls for more 'treatment'. Confidence, or an increased 'internal locus of control' is acquired by being able to do things independently. A further spin-off is that increased responsibility for one's own improvement is more likely to result in the maintenance of any changes achieved.

156

Reinforcement

A physiotherapist's own confidence in the patient's ability to complete tasks is very powerful and hugely underestimated. It was something Brian found very reinforcing. Brian responded well to verbal and non-verbal encouragement and praise. Comments such as 'When was the last time you managed to do that?', 'You have filled that form in brilliantly, it shows really steady work' and 'You certainly look straighter since you have been doing the general stretch routine' helped Brian to feel listened to and taken seriously.

Brian found completing exercise sheets very rewarding as it enabled him to see his daily achievements. Comments made during his admission concerning his poor motivation could now be seen in a different light and tell us more about those making the comments than they do about Brian. With appropriate support and reinforcement Brian started to make considerable changes. (Specific strategies are described in Chapter 7.) However, in order for Brian to continue to make changes outside the department, reinforcement needed to be provided by his family, friends, and himself. Encouraging Brian to discuss with his family what they could do that would help him keep going proved to be successful. Brian suggested that his family use words of praise and help him to problem solve. In this way he felt less isolated, and they were pleased to be involved. He also took up an interest in reading, and for reinforcement his family would buy him a book at the end of each week if he had achieved his exercise and walking goals.

Short term goals

Some simple strategies were used to help Brian start working towards his goals. From the outset Brian was aware that he was responsible for his own progress and the more he was able to apply these strategies the more helpful they would become.

1. **Weight bearing**. The use of scales helped Brian measure weight bearing progress, as even very small amounts of weight bearing were measured and recorded. It also formed a method of self-monitoring that Brian could easily continue at home. He also worked on progressive toe touching exercises, at first on soft surfaces, progressing to tapping, heel contact and then onto harder surfaces. This was made easier for Brian to accomplish by combining with desensitising exercises (discussed below).
2. **Balance**. When building up weight bearing Brian was automatically working on balance, but further exercises and strategies to improve his balance helped him to prepare for public transport and for walking on uneven surfaces. It also contributed to building his confidence about going out. He was also encouraged to reintroduce jolting and altered balance situations—standing on one foot, walking on an imaginary tight rope, and hopping on his left leg. Using these exercises Brian was able to build up his confidence to travel alone and he coped successfully with bumpy journeys and crowds.

157

3. **Walking**. Brian was encouraged to set a daily walking programme. Initially with both crutches, he practised toe touching with his left leg, then walking with one crutch, with two sticks, one stick, and finally without support. He planned this carefully, increments being based on seconds and, later, minutes. Brian wrote the programme down and placed it on his fridge at home, acting as a constant reminder and reinforcer.

4. **Desensitising**. Brian had identified that he wanted not only to reduce the crepe bandages he used but also to improve his skin condition. Following discussions concerning why skin becomes sensitive and why with complex pain problems the level of sensitivity can vary so much from day to day, Brian started a systematic process of applying E45 cream. He started with five seconds over the least sensitive area and progressed over three months to being able to apply cream to his whole leg in a normal fashion four times a day.

Over the same period of time Brian reduced the use of bandages. He did this by removing one of the three for a short period of time, systematically increasing the exposure time until he only used two bandages, then one, then none.

Flare-ups

Flare-ups can challenge any patient. They usually make them think that they have done something wrong and damaging and should avoid repeating it. Brian had previously held this belief very strongly and had had it reinforced by many around him. He needed the information in place to remind him that the increases in pain he would experience did not mean more damage was occurring, that it was common and that it would settle so that he could continue on.

Usually flare-ups are caused by over-stretching (i.e. occur on a good day), under-stretching (i.e. when the pain has already increased for unrelated reasons), or by repeated movements and activities without short rests or appropriate stretching. Flare-ups often occur for no reason at all. Patients need to know all this.

Brian felt that flare-ups made it very difficult for him to continue stretching. With CRPS this is particularly understandable since flare-ups can be particularly intense and difficult to cope with. Reminding Brian that movements if avoided would only be harder to return to proved very helpful, as did reinforcement and encouragement from his family, once they too understood that flare-ups were unrelated to the exercises or to any important damage.

General goals

1. **General**. Brian was encouraged to follow a general upper body strength and flexibility routine, expanding on the weight programme he had previously followed.

2. **Social**. As a result of Brian's pain and reduced confidence he had lost contact with many friends as he found it too daunting to go out a lot. To overcome this, Brian planned a graded approach to socialising more. He started by having friends round to his house, later visiting them at their homes for short periods of time, and building up the duration. He then progressed to visiting less crowded public places and finally returned to watching football games and going to a gym.

Maintenance

The key to maintenance is that a patient develops confidence in his or her ability to cope. The strategies already discussed will help to maximise maintenance. These strategies can be developed most effectively during face to face sessions, but the primary aim of the sessions must be to give patients the ability and confidence to self manage their pain and the problems associated with it.

Telephone sessions can be a useful follow on from sessions in the department. For example, there were times when Brian needed support between sessions and that was provided over the telephone. This helped to reduce travelling and reliance on more frequent appointments but still provided a means of reinforcement for ongoing changes and maintenance. Brian found it particularly helpful to know that if flare-ups arose he had someone to contact. Hence he felt less isolated and so was less likely to seek support from other (possibly less helpful) professionals.

Outcome

Brian changed immensely over the time we worked together. His initial fears and concerns reduced and he was able to work steadily on the exercises. It was not always easy for him as the inconsistent nature of pain and the variety of sensations he encountered often left him feeling despondent and hesitant about continuing. At these times asking Brian to think of what he had achieved and also acknowledging the difficulties he had to cope with enabled him to keep a realistic view of his progress. Both his parents and brothers reported their joy in their more confident person who was starting to look forward and plan.

Brian was seen nine times over a 14-month period, with a follow-up six months later. The initial four appointments were once every two weeks. Appointments were then spread out to every month for three months, then one at three months and one at six months, with the follow-up six months later. At the third-from-last appointment, discharge was discussed and planned so that Brian had some control over when he felt ready to continue working without a follow up appointment.

In comparison to other patients this was a long period of time, but bearing in mind his experiences it was not felt to be an excessive amount of time to work with him. At the time of discharge Brian had not returned to football or college. He walked occasionally with one stick but otherwise was nearly fully weight bearing. He had plans to return to college later in the year and was progressing his gym work. Repeated physical measures were consistent with these changes: Brian increased his walking distance in five minutes from 80 metres to 278 metres, step-ups from 6 to 21, and stairs from 12 to 87 (all without aids) and the circumference of his left calf had grown from 25 to 38 cm.

Discussion

Overall, assessment needs to be seen as an ongoing process. It provides an ideal opportunity for the patient to meet you and for you to gain a deeper understanding of the patient. It is where information is first collected. As you get to know patients and they spend more time with you it can be added to and changed from session to session. Patients may add to information they gave you at initial contact, especially as they gain confidence in your approach and their trust in you develops. Hence the picture you gain needs to be given time to develop. As it changes, your skills will need to encompass this. You are watching a film develop, not taking a snap shot. By employing a hands off, self-management approach, Brian gained the confidence and skills needed to increase his fitness and activity levels slowly and to utilise pain management strategies in the future.

REFERENCES

Countryman KM, Gekas AB 1980 Development and Implementation of a Patient's Bill of Rights in Hospitals. American Hospital Association, Chicago, Illinois.
Patten OD, Nelson S 1996 A preliminary study of patients' perceptions of certain aspects of their physical therapy experience. Physiotherapy Theory and Practice 12:27–38

7

Improving fitness and function in complex regional pain syndrome

SUZANNE BROOK

Introduction

This chapter focuses on the role of physiotherapy in enabling fitness and increased functional ability and how this can be implemented in complex regional pain syndrome (CRPS) utilising the principles of self management for chronic pain. The literature concerning the role of physiotherapy in CRPS is sparse (see Chapter 5), although much that is relevant to chronic pain management is also relevant to this condition. (For further discussion of this area the reader is advised to review Chapters 8 and 9 of Topical Issues in Pain 1, Shorland 1998, 1998a.)

Why exercise is so important

Many patients with CRPS have been told to rest their affected limb or believe that movement will further injure the already damaged limb. This belief is held strongly by many patients and is often reinforced by clinicians. As discussed in the previous chapter, the role and appropriateness of exercise can be confusing for the patient. The suggestion that exercise is important needs to be introduced carefully and backed up with information to help patients understand why it is important.

Exercise needs to be seen as a way of helping patients increase not just their fitness but, more importantly, their levels of activity. Carefully designed exercises enable patients to become active, e.g. to reach for top shelves, carry more shopping, sit on the floor. Activity orientated exercises need to be viewed as being more important than exercises that focus on specific details, like improving physical strength or range of movement. This approach to the role of exercise helps in that it gives patients the opportunity to make the necessary links to their own day-to-day lives. 'What is it you would like to be able to do if you were fitter and looser?' is a critical question. Exercise then becomes less to do with 'What I was told to do by the physiotherapist' and more about 'Exercising will help me in everything I do.' It should not be seen as a chore, something boring and with no purpose, but rather as a means to an end—to be able to do more fulfilling things in life. This in turn helps patients to build up their confidence and enthusiasm towards movement.

Once patients start to move their affected limb even very slightly, their confidence, their self esteem, and their feelings of control and ability to cope with their pain tend to improve. Exercise also becomes an important coping strategy to help manage pain and flare-ups.

The key is to introduce exercise slowly at a pace the patient feels comfortable with and with their least feared movement first. What most helps patients to continue to build their confidence and maintain exercise is the feeling that they are in control of what they are doing. This requires that patients learn to be confident enough to decide for themselves what movement/exercise to work on first and how much to work.

Initially activity goals may not be directly related to the painful limb. For example, one of my patients with CRPS affecting her lower limb wanted to start painting. This did not directly involve the lower limb, but the patient found that when painting her pain increased. This was identified as being due to sitting for too long in one session. By encouraging her to determine her sitting tolerance, and hence limit how long she sat at one session, she was able to progressively build up her total painting time as well as increase her sitting tolerance. She was then able to apply her pacing skills to all activities that affected her pain and function, improving quality of life even if there was minimal change in purely physical fitness.

Exercise has the benefit of reversing many of the changes caused by inactivity and disuse. As long as appropriate information is provided, patients can learn that movement, if done slowly, gently and smoothly, can in the short and long term reduce not only tissue changes caused by lack of use but also sensations such as hypersensitivity, throbbing, tingling and temperature changes.

It is important that patients begin to question their beliefs about movement/pain in a supportive environment and that their beliefs are not challenged directly or harshly by the physiotherapist. Patients should understand that, for example, without trauma a limb immobilised for as little as one hour will start to become discoloured. Upon subsequent movement sensations of tightness, throbbing, and heat may occur. It is emphasised that feelings and sensations like these are normal responses to movement after immobility and not signs of pathology or damage that cannot be changed. Understanding information like this helps patients start to question their own avoidance and fear related beliefs concerning movement and exercise.

An additional benefit of exercise is in the prevention of further negative effects related to inactivity; for instance, loss of strength and stamina, weight gain, and increased discomfort and pain. Information here can be vital in helping a patient begin a gentle exercise programme.

Telling a patient that you are not able to say that exercise will cure them or take a lot of their pain away can be difficult and possibly disheartening. However, most patients when asked whether they feel a cure is realistic for their condition will say 'There isn't one.' 'Selling' exercises to patients who may well have already tried to exercise and found they made them worse, can be very difficult. However daunting this may be to discuss, it is rare that patients are not interested in hearing more. It is important to be realistic about what can be achieved; remember, patients who have had pain for a long time have usually been seen by many different practitioners and are likely to have had hopes built up which later proved unfounded. Thus, patients are quite likely to appear hesitant, negative, or even cynical about the benefits of an exercise approach. Repeated failure easily gives rise to a pessimistic outlook.

From the outset an important goal is to establish the patients' understanding that exercise for CRPS is not about a cure but about helping them gain more awareness of how they can manage the pain and how they can be more active despite the pain. Any change to the pain is then seen as a bonus. This can appear insensitive but unless we, as physiotherapists, are realistic about our role, we only act to set the patient up for further failure.

Exercise, in that it leads to increased activity levels, is of course important for more general reasons, such as returning to social activities, improving general health (aerobic fitness for cardiac health, weight bearing exercise for bone strength, etc.), and the overall benefit of being able to join in with friends and families in such normal things as going for walks, bike rides, and going on holidays.

Difficulties faced when introducing exercises

Every patient comes to a clinician with various beliefs, perceptions and expectations about therapy and about the role of exercises for their particular problem. A patient's previous experience of exercises, and their beliefs about them, are particularly relevant and need to be understood before starting. For example, in the previous chapter Brian had been immobilised for a very long period of time, during which his belief that 'movement equalled pain which equalled further damage' was reinforced. Telling Brian to exercise without acknowledging these beliefs and providing more relevant information could have challenged him so much that he would not have returned for further appointments or might have led him to say that he had exercised when, in reality, he hadn't. This would almost inevitably lead to failure of the approach.

Physiotherapists may be unaware of the subtle messages they may be sending to patients. For example, telling patients to stop exercising when pain increases or telling the patient to use pain level to act as a guide to stopping or doing an exercise implicitly sends a message that the pain is indicating danger or damage and that any other activity that may hurt should be stopped or avoided. Physiotherapists may send a similar message when they change a set of exercises for 'better' ones, implying again that the patient needs safer exercises and that, if done incorrectly, movement is damaging.

Patients will find it more helpful to review with the physiotherapist the way exercises are done. For example, are they slow, smooth and gentle? Do patients need more advice on relaxation and incorporating appropriate breathing with exercise? The ideal message is for the patient to be consistently encouraged to exercise. Technique can be explored and advice early on like 'Do it gently within *your* manageable range and you will not damage yourself' is often very useful. It is also appropriate to reassure the patient that training pain is likely, and that 'rust' may be felt when a stiff joint is stretched. This provides information patients can use to help keep them going when starting to exercise. Here, they now expect some reactions and difficulties, know they are normal, and know that there will be an end benefit.

Experiences after exercise may make continuing with them difficult; for example, if exercises (or other activities) are overdone then flare-ups are likely. If the resultant levels of increased pain become too much it may lead the patient to think that it is not worth continuing to exercise. Some patients will overdo exercise because they believe the myth that there is no gain without pain. Prior to their pain condition the patient may have exercised a lot, pushing themselves in the belief that the resultant training pain is a good thing. If this belief remains a patient with chronic pain will struggle greatly with flare-ups and feelings of confusion and despair. For patients with CRPS, this belief needs to be replaced with a better understanding and flare-ups need to be discussed.

As mentioned earlier, if a helpful link hasn't been established between an exercise and improved function, then completion of any exercise programme will be difficult. Good therapists design and teach exercises so that the patients can see their relevance to a desired goal. For example, a patient may start a lumbar flexion exercise programme with the goal of being able to put on their own shoes or pick things up off the floor.

Patients need to see change and measure it for themselves from day to day or week to week. They also need to have goals they want to work towards and to be provided with the strategies to achieve them (see later).

Where to start

Identify the patient's present activity level

In order to establish a baseline level of activity from which to build it is helpful to establish the patient's current activity/inactivity levels. It is best to find out how active/inactive they are on both a good day and a bad day, so that a rough average can be calculated. In this way baseline activities are easily related to the patient and help to keep discussions more meaningful. It also helps establish what they enjoy, what they avoid, and what they may feel they have to do. It may also act to show patients that they are actually doing some activities despite thinking they do nothing. Asking patients to record their daily activity timetable can be helpful, giving them an insight into what they do day to day and how they go about what they do. For example, are there long periods of rest preceded by bursts of activity or a fixed routine of cleaning days, shopping days and rest days?

The overactivity and underactivity cycle

Patients often cycle from days of overactivity to days of doing very little. This pattern of overactivity followed by underactivity links to days of less pain and days of more pain and can be frustrating for the patient. The danger times are the days of less pain, since patients tend to do more when things hurt less or they feel more confident. The problem is that overactivity and struggling on usually results in pain exacerbation, followed by further rest with its consequences of stiffness and weakness, and the perpetuation of an unhelpful cycle. Pacing and planning are strategies that can change this cycle from continuing, as described below.

Pacing

Pacing is a systematic, incremental approach to building on the amount of an activity or movement that can be managed easily. Pacing is a means to an end, a strategy that will allow patients to increase their fitness and exposure to everyday activities in a gradual way. For example, Brian paced the removal of his crepe bandages over several months. He also paced up his cream application for skin desensitisation (see Chapter 5). Pacing helps patients to change their behaviour from an unhelpful, pain-dependent approach (inconsistent as the pain which controls activity will come on sooner one day and later the next) to a more helpful, time-dependent approach (consistent and easy to measure). Harding (1997) describes the principles of pacing as:

- Make a plan. Prioritise what has to be done on a daily basis.
- Start activities with realistically low baselines, and then build up tolerance to the activities gradually and systematically.
- Take regular rests between activities.
- Change position regularly while performing activities.
- Do small amounts often, rather than doing everything at once.
- Avoid long unbroken periods of either activity or rest.

Physiotherapists can encourage patients to pace appropriately, understanding that there is no rush with increasing exercise/activity levels and that it is the slow, gradual approach that enables long-term change and produces the best outcome. Pacing also gives patients the means to challenge avoided, difficult and feared activities/movements, which can be especially meaningful to people with CRPS. They can be helped to break these down into basic components and then build upon them using pacing (examples will be given later).

Baseline setting

A baseline is the point from which exercises and activities can begin. It is also the amount of activity, which is easily manageable (measured in time or number of repetitions), which can be done comfortably, and does not cause a flare-up in the patient's pain (i.e. pain levels increasing above their normal for a period of more than 2 hours after the activity). Pain which remains high within two hours but for no longer is due to the stretch/exercise being new and can be often be talked about in terms of 'rust' from that movement. The time limit of two hours gives patients something to measure, to help them feel more in control.

Baselines need to be established over several days (ideally two or three, and at different times), thereby allowing for any natural fluctuation in day to day pain levels. Measurements can be made using time or a number of repetitions. The baseline is determined by taking the average of those measures achieved over the trial days and reducing this by 20% (see Shorland, 1998). Thus the baseline is 80% of the average. From this point the patient can decide on the pacing *increments* for each stretch/exercise and activity.

For example, Hilda had had CRPS affecting her right upper limb for six years. She wanted to begin writing again. Her goal was to be able to write a letter to her sister living in America (she always telephoned her). Hilda found holding a biro too difficult so started with a pencil drawing circles. Her initial measures were 12 seconds, 10 seconds and 8 seconds, making her baseline tolerance for writing eight seconds. She practised this for exactly 8 seconds twice a day and built up by increments of 2 seconds a day. Within two weeks, Hilda was able to write joined up words with the pencil, and her tolerance had grown to 36 seconds of writing. Hilda then changed to a felt tip pen and starting writing sentences, building up by five seconds a day. Within a month Hilda sent her sister a postcard. Within a relatively short period of time Hilda had achieved several goals and reinforced her achievements by purchasing a fountain pen! She set her next goal as writing a two page letter to her sister, which she achieved within five months.

Other ways of building up writing could include:

• Paint brush–chalk–crayons–pencil–pen;
• Big strokes–big letters–small letters–small words–long words–1 sentence–2 sentences–half page–full page; once a day–twice a day etc.;
• Greeting cards–postcards–short letters–longer letters;
• Tolerances and baselines also need to be identified and worked up for sitting, grip, elbow and wrist flexibility, and strength.

When anyone starts a new movement or action there is always likely to be some training pain. Patients who have chronic pain are likely to be very reactive and need to very gradually get used to new or previously avoided activities, while at the same time slowly building up their confidence. A sensibly low baseline and a slowly incremented pace will help keep training pain to a manageable level and in the long run provide a much better outcome. Patients often feel that this process of reducing activity or exercises is a backward step and this belief can often be why patients struggle with pacing. Physiotherapists need to acknowledge and discuss with patients that baseline setting and consequent pacing can feel like a backward step but are essential in order for fitness to be built upon and increased daily or weekly. Patients need all this explained in detail, reminding them that if they stopped every movement because of initial pain then they would probably never get moving.

How to build up exercises through goal setting

As mentioned earlier, and as seen with Hilda, goals are a very useful way for patients to monitor and measure their own achievements. By being non-pain focused they help the patient stay within the self-management approach, ultimately with the objective that the patient will become more self reliant. This non-pain focused approach is vital. Commonly, physiotherapists working within a medical approach will gain information about patients' achievements by asking about the pain itself, for example, 'How is your pain?' 'Is your pain better, the same or worse?' If the approach required with CRPS is self management then these questions pose problems, as the aim of self-management is functional improvement and not reduced pain intensity—which usually will not occur. As the patient becomes aware that the physiotherapist's focus is on function and physical goals, they can more readily see change and progress.

Helping and encouraging patients to set realistic, achievable short-term goals for activities they would like to return to, is vital. Goals may be orientated towards work, social, or physical activities. What is important is that they are determined by the patient and not by the physiotherapist.

Once goals are identified, the factors that hinder them need to be determined. For example, Brian wanted to walk more normally. Together we identified what made that difficult: weight-bearing, ankle movement, balance, over sensitive sole of his foot, and leg strength. Brian was then able to work on each separately, then to start putting them together and building up walking as an exercise. By working these out, and breaking down the goals into functional 'building blocks', Brian provided himself with more manageable and realistic starting points for change. Patients can decide, with your support, where they feel confident starting. It is often tempting to think that what has been decided upon is too easy and too low a starting point, but this is a danger area. It is far more helpful to let (indeed encourage) the patient set their starting points too low and then build up easily, rather than set them too high and have to keep cutting back because of increasing frequency of flare-ups and an accompanying sense of failure. The pacing increments (build up of time or numbers of repetitions) can be decided by the patients in daily or weekly changes—the key is that they are stuck to, regardless of whether the patient is having a good or a bad day.

Goals need to be flexible and not cast in stone. It may be that patients change their minds about what they want to do. As Harding (1997) points out, patients need to be flexible in the way they set their goals, learning to alter their expectations and adjust them to compensate for any changing circumstances. Based on the information they have been provided with we commonly see that, as patients get more confident about their future and the things they may be able to do, they set more meaningful goals. Reviewing goals also allows both physiotherapist and patient to reinforce changes and achievements that have been made. If progress is less rapid than planned, it is a point for review, not a failure by the patient (or physiotherapist).

A great difficulty faced by both physiotherapist and CRPS patient is the ease with which flare-ups can occur, even when compared to patients with other chronic pain problems. It needs to be remembered here, that baseline setting and pacing have to be set extra low and paced up extra slowly to accommodate the sensitivity and reactivity of their pain condition. Frequently, maintaining current activity levels can be as reinforcing as increasing them. Patients often feel pressured to increase their pacing continually. Not only may this be overdoing the activity but it implies to the patient that they should always be doing more. It can be very important for patients to be reinforced for what they are doing and that maintaining what they are doing is just as important as building up.

Specific strategies

Desensitising programme

A specific programme of graded touch to areas of altered sensation can help to restore more normal sensations and build confidence about being in situations where the area may get knocked or touched.

Amanda was a lady referred with CRPS to her left arm. She had had pain for seven years. Amanda's arm had become so sensitive that she avoided touching it at any cost. She always covered the arm with close fitting clothes, would not put it in a bath, or go out in crowded areas in case it was knocked. The effects that this had on her social life and confidence are obvious. All this was based on her fears of what would happen if it were touched. Over a period of a month she gradually started to touch it more and return to social activities. She started by touching the least sensitive area (around her elbow) for a few seconds and then increasing the area she touched and then the time she touched it for. Amanda progressed to gentle stroking of the arm, tapping, pinching, touching with different surfaces, cotton wool, brillo pads, and fine threads (tickle), building up to slapping and bumping. Similarly, Brian, described in the previous chapter, found it helpful to use cream as a way of desensitising his leg.

Helping patients with CRPS to gradually and systematically expose themselves to varied surfaces and textures helps reduce and normalise the additional painful sensations they experience. The key is helping the patient

168

to set a realistic baseline of exposure to a new stimulus. One second a day may seem too short to be helpful, but it could be a starting point for someone who has avoided touching that area for a long time. This one second a day could then be increased by a further second every other day.

Proximal to distal

If the patient feels that moving the affected area is too much to start with, or if the exercise results in repeated flare-ups, then introducing alternative strategies into management plans can be useful. Moving joints proximal to the affected area, and doing more generalised movements as opposed to specific exercises for the affected area, can be a very helpful start. Explaining the simple anatomy of how tissues cross each other and how joints link together will let patients appreciate that moving the shoulder will be moving the wrist and elbow, even if it does not seem that much. Encouraging the patient to increase the movement of a proximal joint or area has the effect of enhancing the patient's confidence of the affected areas. For example: introducing pelvic and trunk exercises in sitting or lying positions can help introduce exercises for the lower limb. The use of a physio ball with the patient sitting on it and using balance will stimulate movement in the limbs. If weight-bearing is limited, the duration of exercise on the ball can be set at an appropriate level for the patient. Neck and shoulder exercises help introduce movement to a wrist or hand.

Reduction of aids

Reliance on aids can be reduced and they can frequently be discarded altogether over a planned time frame. Brian successfully reduced the use of both his crepe bandages and crutches through the process of pacing. Brian was clear initially that he felt the sticks helped his balance and allowed him to go out. The latter is certainly true but when Brian was asked to look long term at the effects of using crutches, he acknowledged that they would affect his independence and fitness. Initially it would have been unfair to take the crutches away, but Brian practised walking exercises and as he became fitter he introduced a few seconds of walking without so much reliance on the crutches (see Chapter 6 for details).

Many patients with CRPS perceive that the use of aids decreases pain or protects them from more pain. This is often based on their beliefs and experiences that less movement means less pain. When provided with information about longer term effects such as increased pain and stiffness especially in other joints (Brian's shoulder pain was linked to the use of this crutches), increased tissue sensitivity, flare-ups caused more easily, reduced confidence in moving without support, patients begin to appreciate the benefits of reducing or removing their reliance on aids. Reduction plans need to be done in a slow, paced, and systematic way so that in the long term the patient experiences an increase in independence.

Flare-up management

As with all chronic conditions the intensity of pain associated with CRPS fluctuates and patients will experience flare-ups (increase of pain) and set backs (pain remaining high for more than two days) despite their efforts to manage the pain. Plans to cope with these eventualities are extremely useful and help patients to remain in control of their pain. Patients need to know that flare-ups are normal and will happen despite attempts to prevent them. It is very useful for patients to hear that some flare-ups will arise even when they are doing everything right. Flare-ups are part of the unpredictable nature of ongoing pain. It is important that patients appreciate that the reason for flare-ups are not fully understood but that they happen with all chronic pain problems. (For further details see Harding 1997.)

When to discharge patients

If the criteria for discharge are based on pain relief then patients will either never be discharged or they will be told in some manner or other that nothing more can be done for them. This is obviously not an ideal position for either physiotherapist or patient and is counter to the self-management approach. With the self management approach described here, patients should be discharged when it is felt that they have the strategies to continue working at home. It is often important to agree with patients at the time of initial contact how many sessions you will have together before a review of progress is made. This will not only give the patient a sense that 'physiotherapy' is something that an individual needs to continue with themselves but also gives the important message that they will be learning important skills and strategies to enable them to manage independently. The physiotherapist's role is therefore to help the patient learn these strategies and offer reviews over the longer term. Telephone appointments can be used to reinforce patients if problems arise, but it is best to minimise their contact with the department after discharge.

Conclusion

As with other forms of chronic pain, assessing patients with CRPS and getting them involved in their own functional recovery can be challenging. Some of the major barriers to getting patients more active have been discussed and addressed. It is clear that not all patients with CRPS will be able to make immediate changes to their functional level using a self-management approach. However, this need not prevent discharge. What patients will often have gained is the information and means to start making changes when they are ready.

The self management approach described here, and also in the previous chapter and in several chapters in other volumes of this series, will help patients build their confidence and understanding towards their pain and how they can manage it. Changes that patients with CRPS make will often be slow, but if patients have the right information and strategies they do not need long term physiotherapy to make further change. Hence successful management, in part, depends on the physiotherapist being able to alter patients' measures of success—from unrealistic ones where attempts at large rapid changes invariably fail, to more realistic and modest ones that take time, practice, determination and patience to achieve. What is required is that patients have the information and means to make changes in their own environment, within their own time scales and at a realistic pace.

REFERENCES

Cairns D, Pascino JA 1977 Comparison of verbal reinforcement and feedback in the operant treatment of disability due to chronic low back pain. Behavior Therapy 8:621–630

Harding VH 1998 Application of the cognitive-behavioural approach. In: Pitt-Brooke J, Reid H, Lockwood J et al (eds) Rehabilitation of Movement: Theoretical bases of clinical practice. Saunders, London

Shorland S 1998 Management of chronic pain following whiplash injuries. In: Gifford LS (ed) Topical Issues in Pain 1. Whiplash science and management. Fear-avoidance beliefs and behaviour. CNS Press, Falmouth 115–134

Shorland S 1998a Patient assessment—case history. In: Gifford LS (ed) Topical Issues in Pain 1. Whiplash science and management. Fear-avoidance beliefs and behaviour. CNS Press, Falmouth 135–146

2

Pain management

8

The distressed and angry low back pain patient

CHRIS J. MAIN AND PAUL J. WATSON

Introduction

The primary purpose of this chapter is to consider the application of the principles of biopsychosocial assessment and management to low back pain patients presenting with anger and distress in primary care and community settings. In addressing this topic, a general understanding of the biopsychosocial model of back pain disability (Waddell 1987, Waddell & Main 1998) will be assumed. The chapter can be seen as a further development of some of the ideas presented by Watson and Kendall (2000) in Volume 2 of this series (Gifford 2000). The understanding of the psychological impact of pain and disability as presented here has been influenced principally by the experience of treating and managing patients attending the Manchester and Salford Pain Centre over nearly 20 years. This led to the development of a textbook on interdisciplinary pain management (Main & Spanswick 2000).

The primary focus of this chapter is on management of the individual patient in primary health-care contexts and settings and is derived principally from the aforementioned textbook. Issues specifically of management in occupational settings are beyond the remit of this chapter, but are discussed in two recent sets of management guidelines published by The Faculty of Occupational Medicine in the UK (Waddell & Burton 2000) and by the ACC in conjunction with the Departmentt of Health in New Zealand (Accident and Compensation Corporation of New Zealand 2000).

Presentation with low back pain (LBP) in everyday clinical practice

A number of guidelines have been produced for the management of patients with LBP in primary care settings. In the USA by the AHCPR (Bigos et al 1994) and in the UK (CSAG 1994, RCGP 1996) it was recommended that an initial diagnostic triage be accompanied by a series of management recommendations. These recommendations focus on giving straight forward positive messages such as:

- There is nothing to worry about. Backache is very common.
- No sign of serious damage or disease. Full recovery in days or weeks—but may vary.
- No permanent weakness. Recurrence possible—but does not mean re-injury.
- Activity is helpful; too much rest is not. Hurting does not mean harm.

The overall philosophy of the guidelines is clear.

As far as the actual implementation of the guidelines was concerned, it was recommended that multiple methods might be necessary. As part of the initiative, an evidence-based booklet *The Back Book* (Roland et al 1996), which could be given to patients at the time of consultation, was developed. Some of the principal 'messages' contained in the booklet are summarised in Box 8.1.

Box 8.1   Principal messages in the *Back Book*

- Back pain or ache is usually not due to any serious disease

- Most back pain settles quickly, at least enough for you to get on with your normal life

- Back pain need not cripple you unless you let it

- Your spine is one of the strongest parts of your body

- In most people we cannot pinpoint the exact source of the trouble

- You may have good days and bad days; that's normal

- It's your back and it is up to you to get it going

- There are two types of sufferer: one who *avoids* and one who *copes*

- Be positive and stay active; you will get better quicker and have less trouble later

---

The book appears to be a useful adjunct to management of acute back pain for the majority of patients with self-limiting pain problems who are easy to deal with and who do not make extra demands upon doctors' and therapists' time and resources (Burton et al 1999). However, evidence suggests that most patients attending most physiotherapy departments are unlikely to be acute cases; they are likely to have had their condition for some time (Waddell 1998, Watson & Muncey 1999) and may also have had previous treatment for their problem. Unfortunately, a minority of patients are disaffected, angry and distressed about their previous health-care management particularly if the treatment has failed to resolve their problem or meet their expectations. These patients need more than the straightforward 'educational' approach recommended in the *Back Book*..

The Yellow Flags initiative

The Yellow Flags initiative, with its implications for biopsychosocial assessment and management was detailed in Volume 2 of this series (Gifford 2000). Particular attention is directed to Chapters 2, 3 and 4.

The stated purpose of the development of the yellow flags was to:

- Provide a method for screening for psychosocial factors
- Provide a systematic approach to assessing psychosocial factors
- Suggest strategies for better management for those with back pain who appear at a higher risk of chronicity.

They focused particularly on the identification of a number of key psychological factors:

- Presence of a belief that back pain is harmful or severely disabling
- Fear-avoidance behaviour patterns with reduced activity levels
- Tendency to low mood and withdrawal from social interaction
- Expectation that passive treatments rather than active participation will help.

A number of assessment strategies were recommended and these were supplemented by a guide to behavioural management. Large scale screening, using cut-offs on the Linton and Halden questionnaire (1997), was recommended for situations where it was not possible to carry out detailed clinical evaluation; but for clinicians in primary care or community settings, a more individualised approach was suggested. It should be noted that the applicability of screening questionnaires to the back pain population seen in UK physiotherapy departments often has not been evaluated and so caution has been advised with respect to their use (Watson & Kendall 2000). The associated guide to behavioural management was designed principally for a case-management system in which occupational issues were of major concern.

Kendall et al (1997) also recommended a number of *structured interview prompts* which were to be phrased in the assessor's own words. Each of these can be thought of as a 'stem' question tapping one of 7 key areas of enquiry

(ABCDEFW). These have now been developed into a set of supplementary questions and associated guidance notes to assist physiotherapists in psychosocial assessment and management. They are shown in the Appendix to this chapter (page 193.) It should be noted that the stem questions are not to be seen as 'tick boxes.' They represent issues to be addressed. It is suggested that a conversational rather than inquisitorial style is appropriate in order to elicit the information from the patient. (The utility of this approach and the associated training package is currently under evaluation in both health-care and occupational settings.)

Identifying the 'at risk' patient

The discussion above addressed the use of screening tools to identify groups of patients with potential problems that require the allocation of specific resources, such as within a case-management system or where clinical services are organised centrally over a geographical area. Physiotherapists working independently, however, usually will be unlikely to have much (if any) information at their disposal prior to the consultation. In such situations clinicians will need to use the principles outlined above to identify the important issues and then spend time specifically addressing them. It is unlikely that physiotherapists will have access to previous case notes and details of previous treatment, but these should be obtained where possible. Absence of such notes makes a comprehensive and structured interview all the more important.

In reviewing the history of many patients presenting to the Manchester and Salford Pain Centre, it has become clear that many of the 'chronic pain' patients developed substantial problems soon after the onset of their pain. There is research evidence to show that patients who show high levels of distress early in acute back pain are more likely to remain disabled at twelve months (Burton et al 1995). Further studies are cited in two recent reviews (Vlaeyen & Linton 2000, Linton 2000). It seems likely that had this group of patients been treated and handled in a different way at an early stage, some of them would not have become chronically incapacitated. Box 8.2 illustrates a number of variables that may influence the patient's progress.

Some of these factors are primarily patient characteristics and are dependent upon the patient's beliefs and attitudes. Some reflect outside influences, and others are clearly dependent upon the skills and attitudes of the clinician. If a substantial number of the above factors are identified then it is important to initiate a treatment plan at the earliest opportunity, otherwise the patient may drift into unnecessary disability. Any intervention strategy, however, must be derived from a set of underlying principles and informed by clear and focused assessment. The identification of yellow flags does not preclude the use of physiotherapy techniques of proven efficacy, but the therapist needs to be aware that the efficacy of such interventions is likely to be sub-optimal. Indeed, in the worst cases intervention may fail completely if these factors are not addressed as part of the treatment plan.

Box 8.2 Risk factors for developing chronic pain and associated disability problems

---

1. Patient characteristics

- Misunderstandings re causation (hurt=harm)

- High levels of distress at the onset of an acute pain problem

- Catastrophising (fearing the worst)

- External locus of control (passive, expecting others to cure problem)

- Doctor and treatment shopping

- Substantial anger (at initiating cause, pain itself, and medical profession)

- Fear avoidance of pain and activity

2. Outside influences

- Work, benefits

- Compensation/litigation

- Family reinforcement of illness

3. Doctor/therapist dependent factors

- Unclear diagnosis or mixed messages from different doctors/therapists

- Unclear explanation of pain

- Inadequate assessment or examination

- Unrealistically optimistic promises of outcome

- Reinforcing passivity of patient

- Reliance only on medication or rapid referral

Dealing with negative beliefs and maladaptive coping strategies

By the time patients present to pain clinics and ultimately to pain management programmes they are commonly very distressed and not coping well with their pain and disability. They often develop a very negative thinking style and tend to fear the worst. Such 'catastrophising' is not only not helpful, but also has a major effect on a number of other areas including mood, activity, pain, fear, and anxiety. These characteristics may be present when patients consult the individual practitioner. It is important to point out to patients the likely effects of persistent negative thinking and begin to help them make some changes. Start by getting them to identify the negative thoughts they have and when they occur. Many of these catastrophic reactions are based on a small number of specific irrational fears. The more common of these are presented in Box 8.3.

Box 8.3   Potential fears leading to negative thoughts and coping styles

- Fear of pain

- Fear of hurt and harm

- Fear of future disability (wheel chair)

- Fear of loss of control

- Fear of surgery

- Fear of effect on relationships

- Fear of effect on work

Identify and tackle each of these fears, if necessary writing down the arguments against such fears for the patient to refer to later. Teach and encourage them to stop or block the negative thoughts and begin to develop some positive coping strategies, such as those described in the Yellow Flag behavioural management guidelines (described above).

Enhancing positive or adaptive beliefs and coping strategies

There are a number of simple positive strategies, which may be helpful to the patient. Most of these strategies have been outlined in previous volumes in this series but are worth restating here.

Explain the difference between hurt and harm. Reassure patients about the future (e.g. most patients with chronic back pain do not end up in a wheel chair). Help patients regain some control. For example get them to pace activities, take medication regularly rather than on a pain contingent basis, set small achievable targets for activity and build in a reward for managing well (have a cup of coffee or listen to their favorite CD.)

Many of these strategies may seem self-evident or trivial. They are not. They are vital first step to the patient beginning to tackle the consequences of their pain take control and re-establish normal functioning. By building confidence slowly it is possible to halt the slide into further invalidity and help them to make positive progress either without referral to a pain centre or at least while they are waiting to be seen. A number of specific suggestions for enhancing positive beliefs and adaptive coping strategies are shown in Box 8.4.

Box 8.4 Ways of enhancing positive beliefs and adaptive coping strategies

Get patients to:

- Identify when they are beginning to think negatively

- Identify when they are becoming tense or angry

- Take steps to stop such thoughts and begin positive relaxation

- Change what they are doing when the pain gets bad (e.g. get up and walk around a little)

- Pace physical activities

- Pick achievable goals

- Look at what they have managed to achieve

- Reward themselves when they achieve even small targets

Iatrogenic incapacity

Treatment is not always effective and sometimes it is in fact detrimental. Adverse response to treatment is sometimes termed 'iatrogenic' and is defined as: 'a complication, injury, unfavourable result or other problem which can be directly attributed to medical care' (Churchill's Illustrated Medical Dictionary 1989).

Waddell et al (1984) found, in patients with chronic low back pain, that the amount of treatment received (e.g. bed rest, injections, physiotherapy) was related more to the patients' level of distress and illness behaviour than to the presence of physical indications for such treatment. Patients attending pain management programmes frequently have had a lot of previous treatment, but of all the sources of anger and frustration evident in patients attending pain management programmes, the influence of failed treatment among chronic pain patients is perhaps the most powerful. There are a number of specific iatrogenic influences.

Many patients are fearful of their pain and its significance. Frequently they misunderstand pain, the nature of tissue injury and healing. If such beliefs go unchallenged patients may continue to respond to their pain in an unhelpful way. On some occasions doctors and others actively reinforce such beliefs (more pain means more damage and therefore more pain) by telling patients to 'rest up' or 'let pain be their guide.' Such advice is likely to lead to patients limiting their activity according to their pain. It will reinforce avoidance of any activity that is painful, thus leading to fear/avoidance behaviour. Repeated failed treatment with unrealistic expectations of outcome may reinforce the patient's belief that there is something seriously wrong. Failure to improve may also contribute to the patient's sense of frustration. Patients may also think that the doctor doesn't really believe that they have as much pain as they say, or that it is being implied that their pain is all 'in the head.' If true, this judgement may have been made on the basis of failure to respond to treatment. Such an imputation serves only to make the patients more angry, contributes to their sense of helplessness, leading the patients to focus even more on their pain and seek further opinions. In evaluating the impact of such factors, it may be helpful to attempt to systematise the information available. Some guidelines to systematic assessment are offered in Box 8.5.

Box 8.5 Guidelines to systematic assessment of iatrogenic distress

1. Before seeing the patient, make your own careful evaluation of the patient's records if available.

2. Attempt to distinguish matters of *fact* from *opinions* or *judgements* of other health professionals.

3. Take note of any language used by the doctor which is suggestive that he/she is being dismissive of the patient.

4. Note any symptoms of distress from the patient.

5. Consider the *nature* of previous consultations and any comments on the patient's response to assessment.

6. Try to find out the results of previous assessments and what was actually communicated to the patient.

7. Only then obtain the patient's account of the previous consultations.

8. Evaluate the accuracy of their recall.

9. Try to distinguish their recall of facts from their interpretation of them.

10. Distinguish misunderstandings or confusion from distress (whether anger or anxiety.)

Preparing patients for non-medical approaches

Physiotherapists regularly have to suggest a management strategy where patients are required to increase their function despite pain. Even where there is a treatable 'lesion' patients must be encouraged to adopt self-management techniques that they may feel are irrelevant if they believe in an organic cause. Why should they adopt pacing activity, practice relaxation, or engage in any self management if the cause is a motion segment dysfunction that is amenable to manipulation? Recent research has highlighted the powerful influence of attention, distress, and anxiety on the perception of pain and the response of the individual to it (Eccleston & Crombez 1999) but unless patients can be persuaded that pain is multidimensional, and not simply related to the degree of tissue damage, then it may be extremely difficult to get patients to manage their condition.

Many patients present with a 'Descartian' view of their pain, and believe that the intensity of pain is directly attributable to the degree of damage. They believe that the role of the physiotherapist is to effect a cure. Furthermore, they tend to view the mind and the body as distinctly separate. The 'mind-body' problem must be tackled with care. It is ill advised tactically to begin an interview with a direct challenge to patients' understanding or perception of pain (particularly if they show evidence of iatrogenic confusion or distress). They may already have their own suspicions that if their pain was straightforward it ought already have resolved. Indeed, they may have been offered different diagnoses, 'half-diagnoses,' no diagnoses, or been told that there is no physical explanation for the persistence of their pain (i.e. that it is 'all in their head.')

These issues are not merely of theoretical importance, they are of direct relevance to clinical practice. Physiotherapists, however, must beware of giving mixed messages. They may spend most of the time in the consultation performing hands on treatment and give relatively little importance (with respect to time and rigour) to the non-biomedical component of treatment, other than asking patients if they have been doing their exercises. As a result patients may leave the consultation with the impression that the hands on therapy is the important, if not the only, part of the treatment, thus marginalising the role of their own self-management. The therapist must remember that actions speak louder than words. There is stronger evidence for the value of self management than for passive physiotherapeutic techniques. Regardless of the beliefs and prejudices therapists may have about our own preferred intervention; the primary emphasis of treatment must be placed on the facilitation of self-directed recovery.

A structured approach to the interview which may be helpful is shown in Box 8.6.

General principles of individual pain management in primary and secondary healthcare settings

Good communication is a prerequisite for effective pain management, and a number of recent publications have addressed the subject of miscommunications between doctors and patients (Chew-Graham & May 1999, Chew-Graham 1999). The latter identified not only a wide range of beliefs about back pain in patients attending their GP (perhaps to be expected), but also a wide variation in attitudes to back pain among the GPs themselves. Despite the fact that physiotherapists usually spend more time with patients than do GPs, there has been as yet little specific evaluation into communication between physiotherapists and patients. It would appear

Box 8.6   Preparing patients for non-medical interventions

1. Empathise with their pain. Be sure they realise that you accept the reality of their pain.
2. Share their disappointment that a clear explanation has not been found.
3. Try to defuse iatrogenic distress; talk about the complexity of pain.
4. Explain how we still do not fully understand pain, but that recent research is beginning to come up with newer understandings about what happens in the body after it is injured.
5. Explain that the best way to understand chronic pain is that, for reasons we do not fully understand, the body does not always repair itself properly after injury.
6. State firmly that nonetheless, for most chronic pain, there is no evidence of abnormality in the structure of the body and no evidence of a serious disease.
7. Reassure them that pain is common and that hurt is not the same as harm.
8. Observe nonetheless that when pain persists it is upsetting, can make people anxious and, if sufficiently troublesome, can of course significantly affect a wide range of activities.
9. Remind them that pain, if persistent and severe enough, can compromise people's ability to work, sleep, and perform many activities, including their sex life.
10. Note that if this happens, it is normal for people to become demoralised and depressed with feelings of anger (e.g., 'Why me?') and that they may become irritable and difficult to live with.
11. Furthermore, they may do less and less for fear of hurting themselves further, leading to further feelings of frustration and irritability. Relationships may suffer.
12. Help patients understand that the purpose of pain management is to help people to cope with chronic pain and its effects. The prime focus is not on the cure of pain but on showing people better ways of coping with it, not because they haven't tried or are somehow inadequate, but because chronic pain is extremely difficult to cope with.
13. Place emphasis on showing people how to become more active safely and to recover a lot more control over their pain. Pain management should be thought of as a type of rehabilitation that gives people the understanding, skills and confidence to recover control using their own efforts.
14. Advocate the pain-management approach. It has been shown to be effective in health care settings for patients with long-standing pain and high levels of disability, and is becoming increasingly adopted in the management of patients with pain of recent onset, in an endeavour to prevent them from becoming chronically (and unnecessarily) incapacitated.

that communication is just as important. The emphasis of the communication in a physiotherapy interview is traditionally task focused to identify pathology and will represent the training of the therapist and the school of thought with which they identify. However, whatever the preferred physiotherapeutic alignment, adequate assessment will not be achieved without good communication between the clinician/therapist and the patient. It is necessary therefore to consider the nature of communication in more detail.

Communication styles and strategies

The essence of good communication is the ability to be able to understand the patients' problem from their own perspective rather than from the perspective of the therapist. In order to do this the therapist must gain the patient's confidence. The patient has to be convinced that the therapist takes the patient's pain seriously. Only then will the patient be willing to give credence to what the therapist says to them. The converse is perhaps even more true, i.e. if patients feel that the therapist is dismissive or not taking their pain seriously they will not be prepared to reveal sensitive information nor actively comply with treatment suggestions.

Communication can be considered in terms of purpose, style and content. A number of communication strategies is shown in Box 8.7.

Box 8.7 Communication strategies

- Suspend judgement

- Listen and observe

- Be empathic but not collusive

- Encourage self-disclosure

- Explain what you can do

- Explain what you can't do

- Re-establish confidence

- 'Kick-start' self-control

In establishing a competent appraisal of a patient, the first and most important principle is to suspend judgement until all facets of the patient's difficulties have been appraised. Clinical decision making is subject to bias. All clinicians potentially are subject to their own biases that can cloud clinical judgement. Be prepared to give the patient the benefit of the doubt and listen.

Listening skills are vital. Simply allowing the patient to explain how they feel and asking questions often has a significantly beneficial effect. Predicting what the impact of the pain may have been will reinforce to the patient that the doctor/therapist is not out of their depth but understands their problem. This will help to establish the confidence of the patient. Check the patient's own beliefs about the pain and its causation, correcting any misconceptions at the time if necessary.

Explain the complexity of chronic pain problems and the impact of pain. Give reasons for inquiring not only about the pain but also what the pain has done to the patients and how they have been coping with it. Observe carefully what patients says and how they say it.

Empathise without colluding, as a therapist you must accept the patients' beliefs about their pain and previous treatment, but you must not sanction the incapacity that accompanies these beliefs. Explain that the pain is real. Check if others (including doctors and therapists) have implied the pain is imaginary. Inquire what the patient has been told about the cause of the pain by others. Find out what treatments have been recommended or what they have been told to do or not do. It may be necessary to correct a number of misconceptions.

Many patients are confused having received differing explanations from different professionals. It may be necessary to defuse significant anger about previous assessments and treatments. Explain the potential treatment options with the expected outcome. Explain what cannot be done and why.

For enquiry regarding sensitive information (e.g. use of alcohol or misuse of medication) it will be necessary to approach this in a way that 'allows' the patient to disclose information without feeling threatened. Judgmental statements, aggressive questioning, or even negative body language will not be helpful and are unlikely to reveal the truth. The patient is then likely to become defensive.

Make specific enquiry about their pain, its nature, effects, and how they are coping with and managing the pain. Predict how the pain may have affected their mood (irritability, depression and anxiety), sleep, work, and relationships with others. Explain that this is normal and seen in most patients with persistent pain.

Finally, it may be helpful to consider the content of effective communication. Some key points are illustrated in Box 8.8.

Dealing with distress

Patients frequently show evidence of distress. Given that most patients present primarily with the same symptom (i.e. pain), it is perhaps surprising to find that pain patients differ not only in the intensity of their distress, but also in precisely what they are distressed about. It is very important to establish clearly the specific nature of their distress. This should be appraised systematically and a distress profile obtained which identifies the key features of their distress. It may be helpful to address the issue under the headings shown in Box 8.9.

Box 8.8   Content of effective communication

- Develop and employ competent listening skills

- Carefully observe the patient's behaviour

- Attend not only to *what* is said but also to *how* it is said

- Attempt to understand how the patient feels

- Offer encouragement to disclose fears and feelings

- Offer reassurance that you accept the 'reality' of their pain

- Correct misunderstandings or miscommunications about the consultation

- Offer appropriate challenge to negative thoughts (such as catastrophising)

- Appraise their general social and economic circumstances

- Include assessment and involvement of partner/significant other where possible.

Box 8.9   Establishing the distress profile

- Pain

- Limitations in activity

- Sleep

- Quality of life

- Work

- Previous treatments

In initiating the discussion, it may be helpful to adopt a somewhat indirect approach. Thus, rather than asking if the patient feels depressed, for example, it may be less threatening to observe that many patients with chronic pain feel helpless and find they become demoralised at times. Inquire whether this has happened to them. Thus the patient is 'permitted' to disclose feelings about which they may have felt very sensitive. This strategy enables the therapist to gain a more realistic understanding of the impact of the pain. A number of specific strategies for dealing with distress and anger are shown in Box 8.10.

Box 8.10 Strategies for dealing with distress and anger

- Give the patient time

- Signal that it is permitted to be upset

- Find out gently the particular focus of their concern

- Find out *why* they are telling you

- Identify iatrogenic *misunderstandings*

- Identify mistaken fears and beliefs

- Try to correct misunderstandings

- Identify iatrogenic *distress* and *anger*

- Listen and empathise

- *Don't* get angry yourself

There are many potential reasons for anger and distress. It will be necessary to elucidate the reasons so that they may be tackled. Much anger may be directed towards misunderstandings about causation, and distress at previous management (discussed above.) Sadly, such iatrogenic confusion and distress is not uncommon.

It is a normal to become physiologically aroused when faced with an angry patient, especially when the anger appears to be directed at oneself. Becoming angry or distressed yourself however is not helpful. While it is important to empathise with patients and listen to them carefully, it is also vital to remain detached from their anger or distress in order to preserve as much objectivity as possible.

A summary of the most important strategies in the assessment and management of pain-associated distress and anger is presented in Box 8.11.

Box 8.11 Key strategies for the assessment and management of pain-associated distress and anger

---

- Distinguish *pain and disability-associated* distress from more general distress

- Decide what *you* can deal with and what requires someone else

- Be open about this with patients

- If appropriate, offer to help them enlist additional assistance

- Have a departmental policy for referrals of high risk patients

---

It is important that the therapist identifies the distress associated with loss of function and loss of participation in enjoyable activities. It should be possible to design a treatment plan approach that leads to the resumption of these activities. If this is not possible then acceptable alternatives should be sought. Those patients who make the best progress and become less distressed are those who are able to be flexible in their goal attainment and who have a capacity and identify alternative goals and interests if their usual activities are not possible.

There may be occasions when the issue that is the major cause or maintainer of the distress is not directly attributable to the pain problem, although it may have developed as a consequence of it. Examples might be family breakdown or financial worries. These will undoubtedly affect the treatment outcome, but they are not within the realm of physiotherapy management. In this case the therapist must make clear what matters they can help with, and what they cannot. This does not mean that the therapist is dismissive of the patient's problem. Often all the patient wishes to do is talk to someone about their distress. Every physiotherapist has at one time been the recipient of confidences such as this. However, therapists must be careful not to give the impression that they are able to do anything other than listen and must not intervene unless they have been specifically trained to do so. By informing the patient that you, the physiotherapist, are there to help them with the incapacity and pain, are willing to listen but cannot act upon issues in which you have no training, the purpose of the consultation is clear to both therapist and patient. Physiotherapists are human and feel an urge to help people and may respond to the distress by inadvertently intervening by offering advice and suggestions of ways to cope with non-pain associated distress. This changes the purpose of the physiotherapy consultation and it may be very difficult for the therapist to withdraw such help should they find themselves out of their depth with a distressed patient who is becoming dependant on this approach. The key message is: *Always be clear about the terms of the consultation, what you can and can't do.*

The therapist may then offer to refer the patient for specialist help if they so wish. It is a good policy for physiotherapy services to develop contacts with other departments such as psychology and psychiatry services and to have a policy for cross-referral. This is of particular importance in the rare case of the suicidal patient, and the authors strongly recommend the development of a departmental policy for identifying and handling those patients who express suicidal intent. Although rare, it can be distressing for the therapist to be faced with such a patient without knowing who to refer to.

Conclusion: From theory to practice

Some strategies in planning management

When immersed in the clinical complexities of a significant pain problem, it is important to strike the right balance between appropriate attention to detail and addressing the wider issues. It may be helpful initially to distinguish the patient's beliefs and coping strategies into negative or maladaptive beliefs and coping strategies on the one hand, and positive or adaptive beliefs or coping strategies on the other. The blend within each patient of course is much more complex, but the single-handed practitioner needs to find a way of beginning. One practical problem is the open plan design of many physiotherapy departments, often with only curtains dividing one patient from another. It may be difficult to engage patients in discussing some of the relevant issues in such an environment. If it is possible to perform the initial assessments in a separate room this may assist disclosure of important information. However the authors feel that the physiotherapy profession has some responsibility for ensuring that standards of patient care are improved to a level that such impersonal and open treatment areas cease to be the norm. Outside of the hospital ward few other professions are expected to conduct personal interviews and treatments in such an open environment.

It is possible to help patients with chronic pain and disability problems in everyday clinical practice, even when a full pain management programme is not available. It is essential that all clinicians learn and use the techniques of managing pain patients within normal clinical practice, not only to help the patients with chronic problems begin to self-manage, but also to prevent patients with acute pain problems from becoming chronically disabled in the first place. Much of what has been outlined is neither technically sophisticated nor particularly complex. Perhaps it can be thought of simply as good clinical practice delivered in a humane and understanding way. In their conclusion, Watson and Kendall (2000) offer clear advice about the assessment of psychosocial yellow flags in physiotherapeutic practice (p. 127).

In this chapter it has been recommended that clinical practice can be augmented by specific consideration of the management of pain-associated distress and anger in the individual patient. It has been argued that competent management of the psychosocial component of symptom presentation, in conjunction with appropriate biomedical and biomechanical skills, offers a new style of physiotherapeutic management, perhaps conceptualised as a sort of 'psychophysiotherapy' in which amelioration of pain-associated distress and dysfunction is a key component of clinical management and which offers a framework within which psychosocial obstacles to recovery can be successfully overcome. While it would be foolish to attest that all chronicity is preventable, the evidence is such that incorporation of the psychosocial perspective into the early management of patients appears irresistible. Effective secondary prevention however requires not only re-appraisal of the framework within which pain is understood, but also the development of appropriate competencies in assessment and intervention. Much further work remains to be done.

190

ACKNOWLEDGEMENT

This chapter has been adapted and expanded from Main CJ, Spanswick CC, Watson P 2000 Wider applications of the principles of pain management in health-care settings. In: Main CJ, Spanswick CC (eds) Pain Management: An Interdisciplinary Approach Chapter 18. Churchill Livingstone, Edinburgh

REFERENCES

Accident and Compensation Corporation of New Zealand and the National Health Committee 2000 Active and Working: Managing acute back pain in the workplace. An employers guide. Ministry of Health, Wellington, New Zealand

Bigos S, Bowyer O, Braen G et al 1994 Acute Low Back Problems in Adults. Clinical practice guideline No 14. AHCPR Publication No. 95-0642. Agency for Health Care and Policy Research, Public Health Service, US Department of Health and Human Services. Rockville, Maryland

Burton AK, Tillotson KM, Main CJ, Hollis S 1995 Psychosocial predictors of outcome in acute and subchronic low back trouble. Spine 20:722–8

Burton AK, Waddell G, Tillotson KM, Summerton N 1999 Information and advice to patients with back pain can have a positive effect. A randomized controlled trial of a novel educational booklet in primary care. Spine 1999 24:2484–2491

Chew-Graham C 1999 Chronic low back pain: the interface between explanatory models of illness and medical communications. M.D.Thesis; University of Manchester, UK

Chew-Graham C, May CR 1999 The challenge of the back pain communication. Family Practice 16:46–49

Churchill's Illustrated Medical Dictionary 1989 Churchill Livingstone, New York

CSAG 1994 Clinical Standards Advisory Group Report on Back Pain. HMSO Publications, London

Eccleston C, Crombez G 1999 Pain demands attention: A cognitive-affective model of the interruptive function of pain. Psychological Bulletin 125:355–366

Gifford LS (ed) 2000 Topical Issues in Pain 2. Biopsychosocial assessment. Relationships and pain. CNS Press, Falmouth

Kendall NAS, Linton SJ, Main CJ 1997 Guide to assessing psychosocial yellow flags in acute low back pain: risk factors for long term disability and work loss. Accident Rehabilitation and Compensation Insurance Corporation of New Zealand and the National Health Committee. Wellington, NZ

Kendall NAS, Watson PJ 2000 Identifying psychosocial yellow flags and modifying management. In Gifford LS (ed) Topical Issues in Pain 2. Biopsychosocial assessment and management. Relationships and pain. CNS Press, Falmouth 131–140

Linton SJ 2000 A Review of psychological risk factors in back and neck pain. Spine 25:1148–1156

Linton S, Halden K 1997 Risk factors and the natural course of acute and recurrent musculoskeletal pain: developing a screening instrument. In: Jensen TS, Turner JA, Wiesenfeld-Hallin Z (eds) Proceedings of the 8th World Congress of Pain. IASP Press, Seattle 527–536

Main CJ, Spanswick 2000 Pain Management: An Inter-Disciplinary Approach. Churchill Livingstone, Edinburgh

RCGP 1996 Clinical Guidelines for the Management of Acute Low Back Pain. Royal College of General Practitioners, London

Roland M, Waddell G, Klaber-Moffett J, Burton AK, Main CJ, Cantrill C 1996 The Back Book. The Stationary Office, Norwich

Vlaeyen JWS, Linton SJ 2000 Fear-avoidance and its consequences in chronic musculoskeletal pain: A state of the art. Pain 85:317–332

Waddell G 1987 A new clinical model for the treatment of low-back pain. Spine 12:632–644

Waddell G 1998 The Back Pain Revolution. Churchill Livingstone, Edinburgh

Waddell G, Bircher M, Finlayson D, Main CJ 1984 Symptoms and signs: physical disease or illness behaviour? British Medical Journal 289:739–741

Waddell G, Burton K 2000 Occupational Health Guidelines for the Management of Low Back Pain at Work—evidence review. Faculty of Occupational Medicine, London

Watson PJ, Kendall NAS 2000 Assessing psychosocial Yellow Flags. In: Gifford LS (ed) Topical Issues in Pain 2. Biopsychosocial assessment and management. Relationships and pain. CNS Press, Falmouth 111-130

Watson PJ, Muncey H 1999 The role of fear-avoidance beliefs in short-term response to a graded exercise physiotherapy programme. Poster presented. Pain Society of Great Britain, Edinburgh

APPENDIX

Adapted from Kendall, Linton and Main, 1997)
See also Chapters 2, 3 and 4 in Volume 2 of this series

Initial Assessment Questionnaire

A Attitudes and beliefs about back pain

Stem question

*If someone has had pain for a period of time, they usually have their own ideas of the cause. I know you're not a doctor, but what do **you** think is the cause?*

Rationale

The patient's ideas about the onset and ongoing cause of their pain will influence the credence they give to the physiotherapist's interpretation. If the patient remains convinced that they have one thing, e.g. 'a slipped disc,' and the physiotherapist tells them another, e.g. a soft tissue strain, there will be a lack of concordance about the usefulness of the treatment. This question also attempts to explore the patient's worries that they have not been fully investigated. Issues about not having had an X-ray, scan, or consultant opinion may come up in this section. The aim is to get the patient to air these fears and for the physiotherapist to allay them once the 'depth' of the belief is ascertained.

Supplementary questions

1. *Do you believe that the pain itself is harming or disabling you?*
2. *Do you believe that you are going to have to get rid of **all** pain before you get back to work?*
3. *Do you think that increasing activity or getting back to work is going to make your pain **worse**?*
4. *Do you find yourself worrying in case your pain becomes progressively worse?*
5. *Do you find yourself becoming generally more aware or concerned about symptoms in your body?*

6. *Do you believe it is possible to control pain?*

7. *Do you believe you can do much yourself or it is just a matter of the passage of time or the help that others can give you?*

Intervention

If there are unhelpful beliefs about back pain these must be countered by giving information about the course of back pain, the known causes, the lack of a need for further investigation if a full clinical examination has been conducted. (Note: the clinical examination is part of the process of challenging unhelpful beliefs.) This may be supplemented by giving written information such as educational material. However educational material which gives messages regarding the anatomy of the spine but does not tell people to keep active is unhelpful. The patient's understanding should be checked to ensure that the information given has indeed reduced and not heightened fears. As a general rule ask yourself 'What information do I need to give this person to allow them to move forward to seeing increasing activity as a helpful way to manage their problem.'

B Behaviours

Stem question

What are you currently doing to relieve your pain?

Rationale

This helps to identify the patient's current coping strategy. The therapist should interpret activity and inactivity as indicators of behavioural responses rather than always being indicators of nature of the pathophysiology. Those who are trying to keep active despite the pain, provided they are pacing activity appropriately, are unlikely to have difficulties in remaining active. Extra attention should be paid to those who already are using rest and inactivity inappropriately as a coping strategy and to those who are developing a passive attitude to their pain through over-reliance on self-medication. Patients can be encouraged to identify what they are currently doing, those things they find difficult, and those things that they currently cannot do. From this an action plan for the resumption of normal activity can be developed. Focus on the *positive* things the individual feels they can do and work around that. The above points can be used in developing a graded return to normal activity.

Supplementary questions

1. *Do you find yourself having to lie down or take a lot of rest because of the pain?*

2. *Have you found yourself doing much less?*

194

3. *Have you stopped doing most of your usual activities?*

4. *Have you found it difficult to practice the exercises you have been shown as regularly as you would like?*

5. *Have you found yourself overdoing it on a 'good day'?*

6. *Have you found yourself becoming gradually less active and changing from your usual activities or ways of doing things?*

7. *How bad is your pain on a 10 point scale if '0' is no pain at all and '10' is the worst you could imagine?*

8. *Have you found yourself getting more and more reliant on aids such as walking sticks or other items to help you do things?*

9. *Has the quality of your sleep got much worse since you developed (back) pain?*

10. *Have you found yourself taking much more alcohol or recreational drugs since you developed (back) pain?*

11. *Have you started or significantly increased smoking since the onset of your (back) pain?*

Interventions

This section should be linked in to the beliefs about the cause of their pain and their fears as it is usually these beliefs that drive the behaviour. The intervention identified in that section should be implemented once the unhelpful beliefs are identified. Patients should then be encouraged to see the consequences of their current behaviour. Reliance on rest leads to deconditioning, making it harder in the long term to re-establish activity levels. Patients are encouraged to identify the things they currently can do, those things they find difficult, and those that they currently cannot do. From this an action plan for the resumption of normal activity can be developed. Focus on the positive things the individuals feel they can do, and work around that. Goals for a resumption of normal activity graded should be carefully timed and paced.

C Economic and compensation issues

Stem question

Is your back pain placing you in financial difficulties?

Rationale

Those with a previous history of sickness absence from back pain are more likely to have longer subsequent absences. In the case of access to benefits people may be very angry about the way in which the benefits system has handled them in the past. Denial of benefit may lead to anger and a cynical attitude to other healthcare providers.

Supplementary questions

1. *Have you been hit hard financially as a result of your pain?*

2. *Have you had a lot of trouble getting benefits etc. to which you think you are entitled?*

3. *Have you been dealt with incompetently or unpleasantly when trying to sort out benefits etc.?*

4. *Have you had to get involved in claims or litigation because of pain problems in the past? or*

4. *(Have you previously had back trouble resulting in a claim or in significant time off work?)*

5. *Have you had to take a significant amount of time off work because of pain in the past? If yes, approximately how long?*

Intervention

There is a case to intervene as early as possible in those patients who have history of previous work absence. Leaving it until conventional treatment (analgesia and advice) has failed to improve the situation may be too late. Interventions should be geared to maintain activity levels and encourage early return to work even on modified duties if this is available.

It is unhelpful for people providing treatment designed to overcome disability to become involved in benefit disputes. These can be addressed with the patient by having a departmental policy of openness with regard to access to notes but where the treatment provider does not give additional supporting material such as letter of support for claims.

Most patients suffer financial hardship as a result of work loss and incapacity, few are financially better off on benefits. This may cause additional stresses, for which the physiotherapist will not be able to offer direct assistance. Such patients may require specialist counseling including financial advice or specific debt counselling.

D Diagnosis and treatment issues

Stem question

You have been seen about your pain and been examined. Are you worried that anything might have been missed?

Rationale

Attributions and misunderstanding about the nature of the condition exert a considerable influence on outcome (see attitudes and beliefs above). Patients expecting a passive role in the management of their condition are more likely to become dependant on passive treatments (and on the treatment provider) if this is the treatment offered.

Supplementary questions

1. *Have you been given different explanations about your pain?*

2. *Have you become anxious or confused about the explanations which you have been given?*

3. *Are you satisfied with the previous treatment you have had for back pain ?*

4. *Have you been encouraged to limit your functioning and accept your limits?*

Intervention

This links with the previous question about attributions. The therapist needs to know how those attributions arose, and in particular from whom they came and the level of importance the patient attaches to them. It may be very difficult for a therapist to re-conceptualise the attributions given to the patient by an orthopaedic consultant. It is important to find out the patients' ideas about the type of treatment they feel is indicated. Having gained this information, possible misunderstanding needs to be addressed. This may be very difficult if the patient is particularly fixed on the need for specialist investigation. Once again a full examination and explanation allowing a more benign attribution of the pain problem is the key.

Early patient participation in active management is essential even if this is only adherence to a self-paced exercise or walking regime. Early reliance on passive treatments should be avoided at all costs.

E Emotion

Stem question

Is there anything upsetting you or worrying you about your pain at the moment?

Rationale

It is normal to be somewhat concerned, perhaps anxious, and even upset about pain, particularly if it is severe or recurrent. Stress and worry can affect both the perception of pain and tolerance of it. In the management of musculoskeletal symptoms, it is important first to distinguish *pain-associated disability and distress* from other life stresses. While it may be necessary to attend to both, they must be distinguished.

Supplementary questions

1. *Do you worry that daily activities or work will increase your pain?*

2. *Are you getting demoralised or depressed about your pain?*

3. *Are you becoming more irritable than usual?*

4. *Have you become more aware or concerned about other symptoms?*

5. *Do you feel stressed or feel that things are getting a bit out of control?*

6. *Have you lost interest in your social life or become a bit anxious about mixing with people?*

7. *Have you been feeling useless and not needed?*

Intervention

This may range from simple clarification of issues and re-assurance, to systematic psychosocial intervention (addressing distress, beliefs, and behaviour). Prior to arriving at an intervention plan, it is important to listen to the individual and facilitate their self-disclosure. As part of this it is important to be clear in your own mind what you can and cannot do. At an appropriate time this can be communicated. Since an intervention package is being offered, possible future involvement from other professionals or agencies may be borne in mind but should not be considered at this point.

F Family

Stem question

How does your family react to your back pain?

Rationale

Family members can exert a powerful influence on the patient's perception of pain and disability. It should be remembered that the influence can be either helpful or detrimental. In establishing the role of the family, while the view of the patient on the matter is clearly paramount, it may be advisable to speak with a relevant family member, if this is possible, and agreed by the patient. The physiotherapist needs to form an opinion on whether the family member needs to be 're-educated' about the nature of pain-associated disability and if so, attempt to do this.

Supplementary questions

1. *Do members of your family undermine your confidence and keep reminding you to be careful what you do?*

2. *Are members of your family trying to stop you doing things for yourself?*

3. *Do members of your family make negative comments or ignore you when they see you are in pain?*

4. *Are members of your family encouraging you to try to get back to work?*

5. *Is there anyone you can talk to about your pain and its effects?*

Intervention

Any intervention involving a family member has to carried out with the primary aim of reinforcing positive beliefs, giving confidence to the patient, and encouraging the patient to carry out the recovery plan worked out with the physiotherapist. It may be necessary for the physiotherapist to see the family member separately from the patient to elucidate fears or misunderstandings which they may have, but which they may not have told the patient. The patient can be asked a question such as: 'Would you mind if I had a quick word with your husband / wife / partner? They may have noticed some thing else which may be affecting your pain.'

W Work

Stem question

How is your ability to work being affected by your pain?

Rationale

There are obviously clear limitations on the extent of any influence which a physiotherapist is likely to be able to exert on the work environment. Nonetheless, anxiety about possible work compromise or even work loss may be of major concern to the patient. The physiotherapist, however, must focus on possible pain-associated limitations perceived by the patient. They should determine the extent to which these perceived limitations may be influenced by mistaken beliefs or fears about hurting and harming, lack of confidence in sustaining adequate work performance, or conviction that they can only return to work when they are completely pain free.

Supplementary questions

1. *What do think are the major problems for you in staying at/getting back to work?*

2. *Is work stressful?*

3. *Do you get satisfaction from your work?*

4. *Do you believe that your work is harmful to you?*

5. *Is your job physically demanding in terms of heaving lifting, extended standing, difficult postures or inflexible schedules preventing appropriate breaks?*

6. *Is it a pleasant place to work? Are your workmates sympathetic to people who have pain problems?*

7. *Are restricted duties or graded return to work possible for you?*

8. Do you think that the way back pain is managed at work is satisfactory?

9. Do you think your employer is interested in employees who have pain problems?

Interventions

Try to identify if the person is afraid that their work is damaging them. You will need to find out what they do and how they operate at work (it is helpful to distinguish work task from work style here). Try to help patients identify the work they can currently do, tasks they cannot currently do, ways they can or might get around these, and who they need to speak to at work to enable an early return to work. Find out whether any changes to usual duties are possible. Remember, any such changes to duties must be *time limited* with appropriate pacing to resume full duties as soon as possible.

Reassurance about the nature of their work and offering an optimistic but realistic view of back pain and work is helpful. Suggestions that the workplace, posture or task is the cause of the pain are not helpful. It is almost always better to assist the patient to return to their current work than suggest they make major, permanent employment changes. Finally, direct contact with the employer may be helpful.

3

Clinical effectiveness

9

An introduction to clinical effectiveness

RALPH HAMMOND

Introduction

This chapter gives a brief introduction to one of the hot topics in health care in the United Kingdom. The tidal wave of policy documents flooding hospital departments and clinics asks practitioners to take greater accountability for the treatments they provide. Evaluation of healthcare provision is one of the priorities of the government and this has been given a fair amount of attention in some sections of the media (e.g. National Health Service Executive 1998, Toynbee, 2000). Healthcare practitioners and providers are being challenged about standards of practice, variations in service provision, and which interventions work best. This has heralded the 'third revolution in medical care,' a focus on quality and the effectiveness of healthcare (Relman 1988).

The buzzword of healthcare in the United Kingdom, *clinical effectiveness*, has been defined as:

> The extent to which specific clinical interventions, when deployed in the field for a particular patient or population, do what they are intended to do, i.e. maintain and improve health and secure the greatest possible health gain from the available resources. (National Health Service Executive 1996)

So, being 'clinically effective' involves questioning the results of healthcare in real life situations to ensure that we are:

- getting the most from resources
- putting good research into practice
- using skilled experience wisely
- securing the best health gain possible for our patients.

- It concerns ensuring that clinical interventions are based on the best available evidence under real life conditions. Research may have been undertaken in ideal conditions and so show the *efficacy* of the intervention, but not necessarily whether the intervention is *effective* when it is applied in real life (Mead 1998).

To assess the effectiveness of care, the range of interventions available for a given patient or population should be considered. This should be balanced by an appraisal of the skills required, staff skill mix, and geographical location in which the interventions can be provided. To all this an evaluation of the potential and actual outcomes of this use of resources needs to be added (Fig. 9.1).

Clinical effectiveness

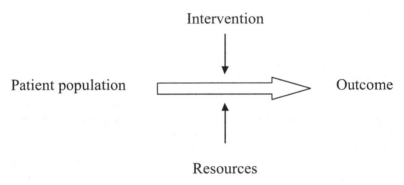

Fig. 9.1 The competing tensions in the clinical effectiveness equation.

Clinical effectiveness

Why do we need it?

Defining quality healthcare is complex, and agreeing how to evaluate how well it is delivered is even more so. Assessment of quality has been conceptualized as involving three areas: structure, process, and outcome (Donabedian 1966).

- *Structure* refers to the resources available for healthcare, e.g. the personnel, buildings, equipment, and the ways in which these resources are organized and delivered.

- *Process* refers to the ways in which healthcare is provided, as well as the behaviour of the patient in seeking and making use of treatment.

- *Outcome* focuses on the results of the healthcare on the overall health of individuals and the population (Donabedian 1966).

While, historically, care has been assessed by considering the *process* of delivery, there is now an increasing emphasis on the study of the *outcome* of healthcare (National Health Service Executive 1997).

The heightened interest in the results of healthcare is based on the growth of the healthcare system, the subsequent need for cost-containment, and the ensuing call for evidence-based decision-making (Van den Bos & Triemstra 1999). With the success of social reform in the early 20th century, and the advances made in medical science, life expectancy has increased. No longer is the result of medicine defined merely in terms of life or death. Society's ability to maintain life has created an older population. It has also meant that a larger number of the community of all ages have multiple impairments and complex disabilities. The success of social reform and healthcare has come through huge financial investment. Expensive drugs, high technology, and human resources have been invested to provide the public with what they now come to expect.

The burgeoning financial investment has alarmed government and created a need for more accountability. This analysis has led to a realisation that substantial variations exist in the use of medical procedures (e.g. Department of Health 2000). In a culture of financial constraints, commissioners now need to compare the outcome of interventions and the qualities of the service provided, and incorporate the findings into their ultimate purchasing decisions.

Little is known of the clinical effectiveness for many health services and interventions (Sackett et al 1996). In the context of cost containment, there is a need to analyse the relative effectiveness of interventions to eliminate unnecessary expenditure. In order to understand the value of a healthcare intervention, the way the care is delivered and the end result of the intervention should be analysed, at both an individual and a population level (Donabedian 1966, Sackett et al 1996). Healthcare commissioners want evidence on effectiveness to help them choose what to purchase, and they are beginning to use evidence of the achieved outcomes to choose where to purchase it (Chesson et al 1996).

Clinical governance has pushed the assessment of the quality of healthcare services by requiring NHS Trust chief executives to have in place mechanisms for continuously evaluating and improving the quality of healthcare provided. This will be expected in private practice. Clinical governance is underpinned by the concept of clinical effectiveness.

Who is it for?

Being clinically effective is of value to everyone involved in healthcare.

- Clinicians need to know they are making the most of their time to provide as good a service as they can for their own job satisfaction.
- Patients want to be treated in the right place at the right time, by the most appropriate person and in the most effective way.

- Politicians have a responsibility to oversee the expenditure of the nation's taxes in an equitable and rigorous way.
- Healthcare commissioners and service providers have to make their limited funds stretch as far as a they can.
- Managers are charged with configuring the service in an efficient way.

What does it comprise?

Clinical effectiveness is the umbrella term for quality issues. It is made up of several elements:

- Evidence-based practice
- Audit
- Outcome measures

When combined, these elements help to assess the extent to which certain clinical interventions get the results predicted within available resources. This process is outlined, simplistically, in Box 9.1.

Box 9.1 How might clinical effectiveness be achieved?

1. Set locally agreed standards for practice, based on the best available evidence

2. Audit the process of delivery of the service against these agreed standards

3. Record the outcome of the service

4. Analyse results of the audit and outcomes generated

5. Change accordingly

Evidence-based practice

Evidence-based practice (EBP) is the 'conscientious, explicit and judicious use of current best evidence in making decisions about the care of individual patients, integrating individual clinical expertise with the best available external evidence from systematic research' (Sackett et al 1996). 'Conscientious' is understood to mean the result of a genuine effort to obtain all literature on a topic, including *all* evidence even when it refutes what we may believe, or currently practice. Just because we don't agree with it, doesn't mean we should ignore it (see Chapter 10). 'Explicit' means having the source of the evidence to hand, being able to cite the reference, and explain where we found it. 'Judicious' means appraising the research in a critical and fair manner.

However EBP is not *just* about using evidence to support practice. It concerns using evidence wisely and integrating evidence appropriately with individual patients. It is a skilled activity concerned with combining the best available evidence with clinical experience to turn the evidence into useful information for a *specific* patient, in *particular* circumstances.

- It does **not** mean that if there is no evidence then we cannot use a particular intervention.
- It does **not** mean that every time a new piece of research is published we have to change our practice.
- It does **not** mean that experience is no longer valued.

What it **does** mean is that if evidence exists we should not ignore it just because it doesn't support what we believe. As a consequence practitioners need to learn critical appraisal skills so we can appraise articles of evidence fairly and make judgements as to the soundness of the methodology, the rigour of the procedure, and therefore the relevance of the results (see chapter 10). It means being shrewd *users* of good evidence, not merely regurgitating the opinions of someone else.

How do you know that what you do works?

Too frequently innovation have been introduced into clinical practice without any appraisal of its value. There are now substantial variations for many interventions in practice around the country. For example the Clinical Standards Advisory Group (CSAG 2000) found that 'specialist services for acute and chronic pain exist in the majority of general hospitals, but there is marked variation in their level and nature,' with some being 'poorly organised.' Not only do patients not get standard treatment for standard symptoms, but also access to treatment and the cost and quality of intervention varies. It is no longer acceptable for patients to receive treatment interventions based purely on the whim of a local practitioner.

By making use of the best available evidence, professionals can reassure patients that the intervention being offered is the one most likely to secure the greatest possible health gain, and that practice is soundly based. This helps to involve patients in decision making, which arguably improves the likelihood of patient compliance with treatment and successful outcome; it also creates circumstances where patients feel sufficiently well informed to choose from the options, and also to decline treatment.

Looking at the evidence

Most practitioners base their core practice methods on pre and post registration education, books, and current customs and fads. For most, there is too much literature to read to keep up to date, too little time to obtain research articles, too many differing opinions and approaches, and a reliance solely on textbooks is of little use as they quickly become out of date. There is now a growing obligation for practitioners to have time to look at and appraise the available evidence. Box 9.2 gives some suggestions for looking at and evaluating the available evidence.

Box 9.2 Looking at and evaluating the evidence

- Focus your attention

- Keep it simple: build your knowledge and confidence gradually

- Find out what's already been done

- Use each other—multi-disciplinary evaluation

- Set yourself targets/SMART goals

One answer to this problem is to look for information that has been systematically found and appraised by other people and to make use of this. This is not new. For years healthcare practitioners have attended courses where experts in the field have disseminated evidence to an audience willing to learn and keen to make use of the results of research. Unfortunately all too often these experts have not been judicious and conscientious with their collation of the evidence and not sufficiently rigorous in appraising the evidence. The suggestion here is that practitioners should maintain a healthy scepticism and be prepared to check the source material cited as well as any other evidence available that may be un-supportive and/or omitted. A generalisation is that for many of our experts, it is rare for evidence to be provided that contradicts the position held. Hopefully as our 'experts' become more aware of the requirements of the evidence-based movement, i.e. that a balance of all the available information is required, their presentations should be of a higher and more trustworthy standard.

Clinical guidelines

Help is at hand. A current fashion is to develop clinical practice guidelines. These are 'systematically developed statements to assist practitioner and patient decisions about appropriate healthcare for specific clinical circumstances' (Field & Lohr 1992). Clinical guidelines are produced to help health professionals and patients make the right decisions about health care in specific clinical circumstances. Clinical guidelines sit alongside, but do not replace, the knowledge and skills of experienced health professionals. **Good** clinical guidelines can change the process of health care and improve the results. They should be written on a carefully defined topic and, after a systematic search, use the best available evidence.

So if we know how the guideline is developed, it should define the search strategy for finding evidence. A good quality clinical guideline should cite all the references used, explain the reasoning for how the recommendations were devised, and provide a grading of the strength of the recommendation and the quality of the evidence. This background information should aim to help clinicians feel confident in following the recommendations made. If a recommendation goes against what is currently being practised, i.e. clinicians are being asked to change their practice, clinicians will, quite rightly, question those making the recommendation and challenge the authenticity of the statement. The worth of a good clinical guideline is in the description of how the research evidence of efficacy has been turned into a recommendation for practice, and this should help clinicians feel confident in applying the guidelines in real life practice.

Research evidence is frequently ranked into a hierarchy. Table 9.1 shows a common classification.

Table 9.1 Hierarchy of evidence

Level	Type of evidence
Ia	Evidence obtained from a systematic review of randomised controlled trials
Ib	Evidence obtained from at least one randomised controlled trial
IIa	Evidence obtained from at least one well-designed controlled study without randomisation
IIb	Evidence obtained from at least one other type of well-designed quasi-experimental study
III	Evidence obtained from well-designed non-experimental descriptive studies, such as comparative studies, correlation studies and case studies
IV	Evidence obtained from expert committee reports or opinions and/ or clinical experience of respected authorities.

Adapted from: A hierarchy of evidence. National Institute for Clinical Excellence (2001)

Good guidelines can be a means for integrating evidence into practice. The value of guidelines is that the evidence has been systematically found, appraised and the results turned into recommendations that might be relevant in helping clinicians and patients make decisions about practice.

However, other forms of systematic reviews of evidence exist. Guidelines are often based on information found from *meta-analyses*. These are the collation of similar but separately published research studies on the same topic and conducted by similar means. By their very nature this will involve quantitative methodologies. The authors of a meta-analysis attempt to homogenize the studies as closely as possible, both statistically and in their analysis, in an attempt to gain greater numbers of patients and so have more evidence on which to generalize the findings, and so be able to extrapolate for a specific population.

Systematic reviews are an approach to collating all literature (qualitative and quantitative) on a specific topic. The results of a systematic review may well be used to inform a clinical practice guideline. Increasingly there are publications that seek to collate systematic reviews. For example the National

Health Service Centre for Reviews and Dissemination (2000) (http://www.york.ac.uk/inst/crd/welcome.htm) summarises the research evidence on the effectiveness of the most common conservative (non-surgical) treatments for acute and chronic low back pain. It provides information on the background to the topic, the nature of the evidence used, a discussion of the evidence, a summary box of evidence for effectiveness, and a section on implications arising from the findings.

As well as systematic reviews and meta-analyses there are other forms of evidence. These can be found in both quantitative research, e.g. randomised controlled trials, controlled trials, and quasi-experimental studies, and qualitative research, e.g. case studies, surveys, and focus groups.

Clinicians should appraise individual articles with caution, as it is unlikely that a single piece of research will inform practice to such an extent that it can be used in isolation from other research on the same topic. To help clinicians develop skills in critical appraisal, protocols have been developed which can, by asking probing questions, be used to steer the reader through a paper, e.g. Critical Appraisal Skills Programme (http://www.phru.org.uk/~casp/).

The culture of clinical effectiveness is demanding a change in working life, whereby clinicians are expected to utilise research and other forms of knowledge to empower their thinking and underpin their continuing professional development. Such activities mark a change in practice by encouraging more time spent evaluating the whole process of their delivery of healthcare. Box 9.3 gives some of the resources clinicians can make use of to facilitate this.

Finding good, reliable evidence and integrating it into practice successfully goes only part of the way to ensuring the provision of quality treatment. There needs to be some system for seeing if the planned treatment does actually occur and also a way for evaluating what the end result of the treatment or intervention is. This is the remit of audit, and is a fundamental part of all professions' practice. It is especially important in healthcare where intervention can vary so widely, and the difference between effective and ineffective treatment so devastating.

Audit

Audit is a way of measuring the quality of healthcare provided by a service: performance is measured against pre-set standards. The results of an audit are then analysed. This should help to identify where changes are needed. Success in clinical audit is indicated by improvements in the quality of care for patients.

How does audit help?

Audit is a means of providing feedback to frontline clinicians; it shows the results of what they have been doing, comparing them to what was planned. In the rush of daily practice it can be hard to accurately reflect and consider the impact of practice because all too soon another patient comes along.

Audit can also provide managers and commissioners with information about how successfully resources are being used. This can help base decisions on skill mix, professional development, and organisation of service delivery.

Box 9.3 Some sources of collated evidence and help for clinical practice

---

1. Hospital library/librarian

2. Electronic databases: Cochrane Database of Systematic Reviews, web site: http://www.update.com/Cochrane/default.HTM

3. Database of Abstracts of Reviews of Effectiveness (DARE), web site: http://agatha.york.ac.uk/darehp.htm

4. Published literature summaries, e.g. Effective Health Care Bulletins, web site: http://www.york.ac.uk/inst/crd/ehcb.htm

5. Government initiatives:

   The National Electronic Library for Health, web site: http://www.nelh.nhs.uk/

   The National Institute for Clinical Excellence, web site: www.nice.org.uk

6. Clinical effectiveness facilitators/audit officers

The process of audit requires standards for a specific topic to be agreed; this can be at a national or local level. These standards will determine the agreed quality for the specific topic. The service is then provided for an agreed period, after which auditors compare actual performance against the predetermined plan.

The value in the process of audit then lies in considered analysis of the findings and subsequent feedback to the clinicians. This is vital if lessons from the audit are to be learnt, and the process is not to be seen as a paper exercise.

Audit is a useful way for evaluating the *process* of care. Outcome measures are a means of talking about the *results* of healthcare in terms of how much change has occurred.

Outcome measures

A physical therapy outcome measure is a 'test or scale administered and interpreted by physical therapists that has been shown to measure accurately a particular attribute of interest to patients and therapists and is expected to be influenced by intervention' (Mayo 1994). Measures should record change, and show the difference from one point in time (usually before an intervention) to another point in time (usually following an intervention)

(Kendall 1997). It is therefore vital that clinicians record the outcome of treatment at a point in time when they are expecting the effect of treatment to have occurred. This might not be on a sessional basis; it may take several weeks or months for the true effect of treatment to occur.

Healthcare professionals have long been encouraged to use outcome measures as part of the process of evaluating their practice (e.g. Partridge 1982). However the type of information required in pain rehabilitation is extremely difficult to capture. X-rays, blood tests, and scans alone don't provide the whole picture. Much of what is recorded is information primarily from what the patient reports ('My pain has gone') or from observed behaviour. This **subjective** information is difficult to record succinctly in order to contain the time spent making records, however it **needs** to be recorded.

An outcome measure should be standardized, with explicit instructions for administration and scoring (McDowell & Newell 1996 p 494). How it should be administered must be explained, and this requires careful wording to avoid misinterpretation. Ideally, a measure should be reliable, valid, and responsive to clinical change that occurs over time (Binkley et al 1999). However no measure will ever be perfect in fulfilling these criteria. **Reliability** is concerned with how the test can be repeated uniformly when administered on more than one occasion or by more than one rater. A measure may have been tested for reliability, but it is vital that whoever administers the measure does so in a consistent way otherwise the most reliable measure is rendered useless. **Validity** has to do with the extent to which the measure records what it intends to measure, i.e. whether it is asking the right questions (Cole et al 1994). The validity of a measure will depend upon the location it is to be used in and the population it will be used with. **Responsiveness** is the ability of the measure to detect true change in patients' status over time (Binkley et al 1999). Is it sensitive to the subtle changes patients make?

Measures should be convenient for use by clinicians and especially convenient for the patient. In this respect they need to be comfortable and painless, short, simple, and easy to use. There is a constant tension between finding a measure that is short and simple for routine clinical use, and ensuring that it will provide sufficient information that picks up the changes a patient makes. Who the information is really for will help determine the level of sensitivity required.

Attribution

The results obtained with a measure should be analysed to see whether the recorded change in health status is attributable to the intervention. In order to make rational decisions about whether an intervention is of value, judicious analysis of the cause of the outcome should be made (Sackett et al 1996).

Continuing professional development

Much of what clinical effectiveness is about is not new. What is different is how we respond to a more intensive environment to act smarter. To respond to these pressures and challenges, healthcare professionals need to refine their means for managing information. This response should recognise that there are many different ways of learning, more than merely attending weekend courses, and build strategies to optimise learning into their working life. This requires guidance from managers and those in charge, and mutual peer support to give confidence and encouragement and time for constructive and active reflection of practice in working hours.

Conclusion

Healthcare providers and practitioners are being challenged to analyse the outcome of care like never before. Clinical effectiveness considers the extent to which interventions achieve their goals. At present this is difficult to assess as far too little is known of the results of many health services and interventions.

Being clinically effective requires getting the best from the resources available through genuine inter-professional collaboration, use of best practices from other parts of the country, integration of good research, and a sincere desire to integrate individual patients' values and beliefs into their care. The concept aims to improve patient outcomes and public accountability by providing value for money and a return on the research investment. Therapists must act on and be aware of the available options. Also, by really being included in the decision making process, patients should receive more timely and appropriate interventions.

REFERENCES

Binkley JM, Stratford PW, Lott SA et al 1999 The lower extremity functional scale (LEFS): Scale development, measurement properties, and clinical application. Physical Therapy 79(4):371–383

Brettle AJ et al 1998 Searching for information on outcomes: do you need to be comprehensive? Quality in Healthcare 7:163–167

Bruton A, Conway JH, Holgate ST 2000 Reliability: what is it, and how is it measured? Physiotherapy 86(2): 94–99

Bury T, Mead J (eds) 1998 Evidence-based Healthcare. Butterworth-Heinemann, London

Chesson R, Macleod M, Massie S 1996 Outcome measures used in therapy departments in Scotland. Physiotherapy 82(12):673–679

Clinical Standards Advisory Group 2000 Services for Patients with Pain. Department of Health, London

Cole B et al 1994 Physical Rehabilitation Outcome Measures. Canadian Physical Therapy Association, Ontario

Department of Health 1997 The New NHS—Modern, Dependable: A national framework for assessing performance. HMSO, London

Department of Health 2000 The National Plan. HMSO, London

Deyo RA, Battie M, Beurskens AJHM et al 1998 Outcomes measures for low back pain research. Spine. 23(18):2003–2013

Donabedian A 1966 Evaluating the quality of medical care. Mill Mem Fund Quart. 44 (2):166–206

Field MJ, Lohr KN 1992 Guidelines for Clinical Practice: From Development to Use. National Academy Press, Washington DC

Kendall N 1997 Developing outcome assessments: A step by step approach. New Zealand Journal of Physiotherapy Dec:11–17

Mayo N 1994 Outcome measures or measuring outcome. Physiotherapy Canada. 46 (3):145–147

McDowell I, Newell C 1996 Measuring Health—A guide to rating scales and questionnaires. Oxford University Press, Oxford

National Health Service Centre for Reviews and Dissemination 2000 Acute and Chronic Low Back Pain. Effective Healthcare Bulletin, University of York

National Health Service Executive 1996 Promoting Clinical Effectiveness: A framework for action in and through the NHS. HMSO, London

National Health Service Executive 1997 The New NHS—Modern and dependable. Department of Health, HMSO, London

National Health Service Executive 1998 A First Class Service—Quality in the new NHS. Department of Health, HMSO, London

Partridge C J 1982 The outcome of physiotherapy and its measurement. Physiotherapy. 68(11):362–363

Relman AS 1988 Assessment and accountability: The third revolution in medical care. New England Journal of Medicine 319(18):1220–1222

Roos EM, Roos HP, Lohmander LS et al 1998 Knee injury and osteoarthritis outcome score (KOOS)—development of a self-administered outcome measure. Journal of Sports Physical Therapy 78(2):88–96

Sackett DL, Rosenburg WM, Gray MJA et al 1996 Evidence-based medicine: What it is and what it isn't. British Medical Journal 312:71–72

Toynbee P 2000 A good prognosis. The nation's health: Tony Blair pins his credibility on a dramatic modernisation of the NHS. Friday March 24, The Guardian. London

Van den Bos GAM, Triemstra AHM 1999 Quality of life as an instrument for need assessment and outcome assessment of health care in chronic patients. Quality in Health Care 8:247–252

10

TENS and acupuncture for chronic pain: where's the evidence?

LESLEY SMITH

Introduction

Healthcare professionals have ever-increasing amounts of information to read and digest merely to keep up with new research findings. Individual trials often give conflicting results, and it can be almost impossible to assimilate and assess all of the available information on a particular topic given the usual constraints on time. Systematic reviews aim to overcome some of these difficulties by bringing together all of the available evidence, and at their best, provide clear, evidence-based statements about the efficacy and adverse effects of treatments, and where possible, how different treatments compare. This chapter aims to introduce the reader to the basic principals of the systematic review process, and then apply these to appraising the evidence of acupuncture and transcutaneous electrical nerve stimulation (TENS) for effective pain relief.

A systematic review can be defined as a review of a particular subject undertaken in such a way that the risk of bias is reduced. This involves searching for all published and sometimes unpublished information on a topic, appraising the quality of individual studies to determine which studies meet pre-defined inclusion criteria, extracting appropriate outcome data and analysing the results (Fig. 10.1). Reviews done in a non-systematic way or that are selective in the studies chosen may lead to biased conclusions.

Many lessons have been learned over the last few years about what aspects of clinical trial design are important in order to eliminate bias. To determine the effectiveness of interventions such as drugs, the best evidence comes from large, well-designed, randomised controlled trials (RCTs) that are double blind. However, there are other aspects of clinical trial design that are important for scientific rigour. If trials have methodological weaknesses

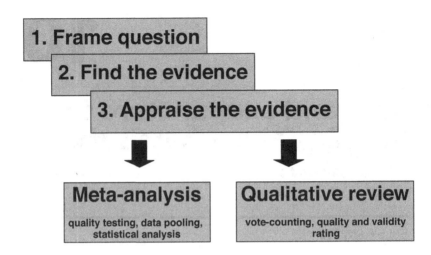

Fig. 10.1 The systematic review process.

then the results are not robust. A systematic review is only as good as the individual trials included. The gold standard for any review is to include the highest quality evidence available to answer the question.

Common sources of bias

Lack of randomisation is a major source of bias in trials. Randomisation overcomes selection bias that can lead to over-estimation of treatment effects by as much as 40% (Schultz 1995). Adequate randomisation ensures that each patient has the same chance of receiving each treatment and the investigators cannot predict which treatment was given. Restricting systematic reviews to include only randomised studies therefore makes sense for reviews of treatment effectiveness. In some situations randomisation of patients to different treatment groups is not possible, e.g. in palliative care, however, this does present difficulties in drawing conclusions from the results. Non-randomised studies are subject to bias and should be interpreted with caution.

Adequate blinding of the study is necessary to overcome observer bias. To be described as double blind, neither the patient nor trial investigators should be able to identify the treatment being assessed. Studies that are not blind may overestimate treatment effects by as much as 17% (Schultz 1995). For many non-drug interventions, blinding is difficult. Some of these difficulties can be overcome by ensuring that at the very least trials are single blind by the use of an investigator collecting the outcome data unaware (blinded) of the treatment received.

Trials with small group sizes are unreliable (Moore et al 1998). As a yardstick, in an RCT of a typical effective drug given for acute postoperative pain, approximately 50% of the patients in the active drug group, and 20% in the inactive drug group (placebo) will report effective pain relief (Collins et al 1998). In this case, to be 95% confident that a statistically significant difference could be demonstrated, at least 40 patients per group would be needed. Many trials of alternative/complementary therapies have less than 40 patients per group. It is important to consider whether failure to demonstrate a statistical significant difference is due to lack of effect or lack of data. For RCTs of analgesics, even with 40 patients per treatment group, the random play of chance can have a significant impact on the result. Figure 10.2 shows all randomised, double blind, placebo-controlled trials of aspirin 600/650 mg for acute post-operative pain (Edwards et al 1999). The trials were conducted under similar circumstances; all patients underwent an operation involving an incision, pain was of at least moderate intensity before the study drug was taken, and pain was measured using identical pain relief or pain intensity scales for four to six hours after the study start. The outcome for each trial is the number of patients achieving at least 50% pain relief with drug or placebo derived using validated equations (Moore 1996, Moore 1997a, Moore 1997b). The variability across trials in the number of patients achieving the outcome in both drug and placebo groups ranges from 1–90% (mean 40%) for aspirin 600/650 mg, and from 0–50% (mean 17%) for placebo. This variability is not unique to aspirin or indeed to trials with a subjective outcome such as pain, but is also a feature of other therapeutic areas such as anti-emetics for vomiting and smoking cessation with nicotine replacement therapy. Computer modelling of 10,000 simulated trials shows that the variation is largely due to the random play of chance on group sizes of about 40 patients (Moore et al 1998). Large numbers are needed to overcome this. The country a trial is conducted in can also be a source of bias. Of controlled trials of acupuncture conducted in Asia and former Soviet countries, almost all (91–100%) were positive compared with 60% of those conducted in Western Europe, Australasia, or North America (Vickers et al 1998). This relationship was also true for treatments other than acupuncture. There may be valid reasons for these differences in trial outcome, but care should be taken when interpreting the results of these trials or reviews as they may represent differences in trial conduct.

Trials included in systematic reviews of acupuncture and TENS may have some of these shortcomings. But if those are the only trials available to the reviewer then she is faced with evaluating them. As long as the trials are interpreted with caution and appropriate weight placed on their findings this should not be a problem.

Transcutaneous electrical nerve stimulation (TENS)

TENS is a method of pain relief based on the gate theory and is widely used by physiotherapists for acute and chronic pain conditions. Systematic reviews of TENS for postoperative pain (Carroll et al 1996) and TENS for chronic

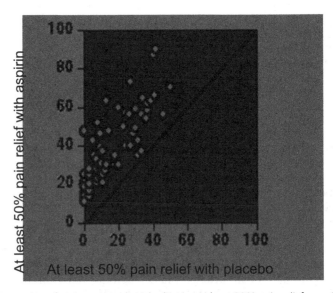

Fig. 10.2 Proportion of patients in each trial achieving at least 50% pain relief over 4–6 hours with aspirin 600/650 mg versus placebo. Each circle on the plot represents the results of an individual trial. Read the plot the same as any graph where the co-ordinates represent the location of the circle on the plot (e.g. if in a trial 20% achieve 50% pain relief with placebo and 50% with the drug a circle would be above the line at 50% on the y axis and 20% across on the x axis.) The reason all of the circles are above the line of equality is because in all of the trials the drug was more effective than placebo.

pain (McQuay & Moore 1998) have been conducted. A summary of the findings of these systematic reviews may also be found on the Oxford Pain Internet site at: www.ebandolier.com.

TENS for chronic pain

All published RCTs that compared TENS to placebo (sham TENS) or active treatment groups (NSAIDs) of patients with chronic pain, and reported on pain outcome measures, were sought and assessed (McQuay & Moore 1998). Blinding of TENS for patients and anyone involved in the trial is particularly difficult and none of the trials was considered adequately blinded, though attempts were made by most. Twenty-four trials compared TENS with placebo (sham TENS); of these 10 reported a statistically significant difference on at least one pain outcome and thus were judged positive. Fifteen trials used an active control group, of which three reported a positive outcome. The overall conclusion drawn from these trials is that they represent lack of evidence of effect rather than evidence of lack of effect. Many of the negative studies failed to detect a statistically significant difference between TENS and placebo. This may be due to inadequate dose and duration of treatment, or inadequate number of patients. Previous studies have recommended TENS treatment for 30 minutes twice a day for at least a month for chronic pain relief (Johnson et al 1992). In most of the studies TENS was given for shorter treatment periods than this. The use of TENS for chronic pain may well be justified, but the evidence does not support this at present.

TENS for acute pain

This systematic review set out to determine the importance of randomisation in controlled trials of TENS for acute postoperative pain (Carroll et al 1996). All controlled trials, randomised and non-randomised, comparing TENS with placebo or active controls for acute postoperative pain and reporting pain outcome measures were sought. Seventeen RCTs compared TENS with placebo; of these 15 failed to show a statistically significant difference between the two treatment groups. Nineteen non-randomised controlled trials were found; in 17 TENS was judged to have had a positive analgesic effect by their authors (Fig. 10.3). These data clearly illustrate the importance of randomisation in trials with pain outcome measures. The inclusion of non-randomised studies may lead to erroneous conclusions.

Both of these reviews are examples of qualitative systematic reviews where a final vote counting exercise, how many positive, versus how many negative trials, is used to determine whether the intervention is effective or not. A weakness of this method is that it is based on each trial's own estimate of positive or negative and takes no account of how valid the estimate is. For example, it does not take into consideration the size of the trial or the size of the effect, so that a small trial with a bare statistically significant positive result would have the same weight as a large trial that showed a conclusive negative. This is in contrast to quantitative systematic reviews (meta-analyses) where pooling of data at least weights trial size and effect size. One way of overcoming this weakness is to take the validity of each trial into consideration, and to give more weight to the trials of highest validity when drawing an overall conclusion.

There is no single recognised way of assessing trial validity. However, we know that trials can report inaccurate or misleading results when the methodology is biased or inadequate. Double blind trials with large groups, validated outcome measures, sensitive designs and appropriate methodologies are less biased than those without. An example of a systematic review that includes an assessment of trial validity, is one of acupuncture for back and neck pain (Smith et al 2000) and is summarized below.

Acupuncture for back and neck pain

All published RCTs that compared acupuncture with placebo (sham acupuncture, sham TENS, no treatment or waiting list) and reporting pain outcome measures were sought. Thirteen RCTs were included and summarized as a qualitative systematic review. Data pooling for meta-

	Analgesic effect	
	Positive	**Negative**
Randomised	2	15
Inadequate or not randomised	17	2

Fig. 10.3 TENS for postoperative pain.

analysis was not possible due to differences in treatment regimes, patient characteristics, control groups, outcome measures and trial design. The included trials were assessed for quality and validity using The Oxford Pain Validity Scale (OPVS) (Smith et al 2000). The OPVS was designed to evaluate aspects of trial methodology known to be sources of bias in RCTs of pain interventions and consists of five items: blinding status, group size, outcome measures, baseline pain, and trial sensitivity and data analysis (Table 10.1). For each trial, a score is assigned from 0–16, the higher the score the more valid the result. This enabled more weight to be placed on the trials of higher quality and validity in drawing an overall conclusion about the efficacy of acupuncture for back and neck pain.

What is the evidence that these items are important in pain trials?

- **Blinding**. A trial should be adequately blinded to eliminate observer and patient bias. Blinding is especially important when outcomes are subjective (e.g. pain, nausea) rather than objective (e.g. death, vomiting).
- **Group size**. Trials with small group sizes are unreliable (Moore et al 1998). As a yardstick, a typical effective treatment for acute or chronic pain has an analgesic response rate of approximately 50%, and placebo response rate of 20% for an outcome of pain half gone. In this case, to be 95% confident that a statistically significant difference could be demonstrated, at least 40 patients per group would be needed.
- **Outcome measures**. Poor outcome measures give unreliable findings. Standard pain intensity or pain relief measures, rated by the patient, are the most reliable estimate of efficacy (Moher et al 1995). Outcome measures assessed by the physician or carer may over-estimate treatment effect (Rundshagen et al 1999). Analgesic consumption is not a sensitive measure of pain relief.
- **Baseline pain**. A trial with no or little pain at baseline cannot measure a reduction.
- **Internal sensitivity**. A trial that cannot demonstrate that it is sensitive enough to measure an effect is of limited validity. Does a negative result

Table 10.1 The Oxford Pain Validity Scale (OPVS)

Item		Score (circle one number per item)
Blinding	1. Was the trial convincingly double-blind?	6
	2. Was the trial convincingly single-blind?	3
	3. Was the trial either not blind or the blinding was unclear?	0
Size of the trial groups	1. Was the group size ≥40?	3
	2. Was the group size 30 to 39?	2
	3. Was the group size 20 to 29?	1
	4. Was the group size 10 to 19?	0
Outcomes	Look at outcomes relevant to the review question:	
	1. Did the trial include standard outcome measures, and use the outcome appropriately?	2
	2. Did the trial include non standard outcomes and/or use the outcome inappropriately?	0
Baseline pain and internal sensitivity	1. For all treatment groups, baseline levels were sufficient for the trialist to measure a change following the intervention (i.e. there was enough baseline pain to detect a difference between baseline and post-treatment levels). Alternatively, did the trial demonstrate internal sensitivity?	1
	2. For all treatment groups, baseline levels were insufficient to be able to measure a change following the intervention, or baseline levels could not be assessed, or internal sensitivity was not demonstrated.	0
Data analysis	**Definition of outcomes**	
	1. Did the paper define the relevant outcomes clearly, including where relevant, exactly what 'improved', 'successful treatment', etc represented?	1
	2. Did the paper fail to define the outcomes clearly?	0
	Data presentation: location and dispersion	
	1. Did the paper present either mean data with standard deviations, or median with range or dichotomous outcomes, or sufficient data to enable extraction of any of these?	1
	2. Did the paper fail to present the above?	0
Statistical testing	1. Did the trialist choose an appropriate statistical test, with correction for multiple tests where relevant?	1
	2. Did the trialist choose inappropriate statistical tests and/or multiple testing was carried out, but with no correction, or, no statistics were carried out.	0
Handling of dropouts	1. Was the dropout rate either ≤10%, or, was it >10% but dropouts were included in an intention-to-treat analysis.	1
	2. Was the dropout rate >10% and dropouts were not included in the analysis, or, it was not possible to calculate a dropout rate from data presented in the paper?	0

mean the intervention does not work, or that the trial failed to measure the effect? For trials that do not have a placebo group, an additional active control group of an intervention with proven efficacy is an important way of demonstrating that the trial is sensitive enough to measure an effect.

- **Definition of outcomes.** A trial with unclear definitions of outcomes such as 'clinical improvement' or 'successful treatment' is less valid than one with clear definitions.
- **Presentation of data.** Papers should support their findings by presenting mean or median data with dispersion values (standard deviation, interquartile range) or dichotomous data. Without this information it is difficult to see how authors have reached their conclusions.
- **Statistical tests.** Reports should choose the correct tests, not do too many of them (data trawling), and correct for multiple testing. Any single statistical significance that is the result of multiple testing, and that emerges among many negatives, lacks credibility.
- **Handling of drop-outs.** A trial that does not report drop-out rates, or does not adequately handle drop-outs in the efficacy analysis, is less valid. Studies may lose patients for many different reasons. Unless high dropout rates make good clinical sense, a rule of thumb can be that when the proportion of lost patients and data exceeds 10%, the validity of the data declines unless an intention-to-treat analysis has been used.

Trials were generally of low quality with many methodological flaws including, lack of blinding, small group sizes, poorly defined outcome measures and lack of statistical rigour. The duration and type of acupuncture treatments varied and included single and multiple sessions, traditional Chinese acupuncture, manual, electrical or laser stimulation. Based on a vote counting exercise, five trials concluded that acupuncture provided better pain relief than placebo and eight that it did not. Does this mean that the intervention works? In a simple vote-counting exercise, it would be difficult to draw a conclusion. However, when trials were ranked according to validity, it was found that the more valid trials were less likely to show a positive finding (Fig. 10.4). The overall conclusion was that there is no convincing evidence that acupuncture is more effective than placebo for neck or back pain.

A number of systematic reviews of acupuncture for different pain conditions have been published. Some of these suggest that acupuncture is effective for a variety of conditions (e.g. migraine and dental pain). When the trials included in the systematic reviews are examined in greater detail, a general pattern emerges. The trials showing a positive benefit of acupuncture have methodological weaknesses leading to major sources of bias. The higher quality studies overwhelmingly failed to demonstrate a difference between acupuncture and placebo (Ezzo 2000). A number of these systematic reviews have been summarised for the Bandolier Alternative Therapy website. They can be accessed at: www.ebandolier.com/.

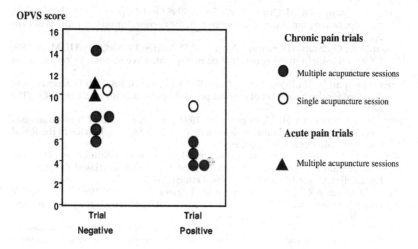

Fig. 10.4 Acupuncture for back or neck pain. Distribution of validity scores using OPVS and overall trial findings.

Conclusion

Critics of evidence based medicine (EBM) and systematic review cite the shortcomings of RCTs not reflecting the characteristics and conditions in which they work. It is often said that patients recruited into RCTs don't represent the kind of patients seen in clinical practice, and therefore the results are not generalisable. Another criticism is that EBM is often seen as a dogma and leaves no room for professional experience and judgement. It should be thought of as a tool to aid clinical decision-making and not as a rule to follow blindly. Whilst there is little evidence to support the efficacy of acupuncture and TENS for chronic pain conditions, there may be patients who benefit from them.

For acupuncture and TENS there is a need for randomised controlled trials conducted to a high quality, with adequate numbers of patients and standard pain outcome measures. Without evidence these potentially valuable interventions may be under-used, or ineffective interventions may remain in use.

REFERENCES

Carroll D, Tramer M, McQuay H, Nye B, Moore A 1996 Randomization is important in studies with pain outcomes: systematic review of transcutaneous electrical nerve stimulation in acute postoperative pain. British Journal of Anaesthesia 77(6):798–803

Collins SL, Moore RA, McQuay HJ, Wiffen PJ 1998 Oral ibuprofen and diclofenac in post-operative pain: a quantitative systematic review. European Journal of Pain 2(4):285–291

Edwards JE, Oldman AD, Smith LA, Carroll D, Wiffen PJ, McQuay HJ, Moore RA 1999 Oral aspirin in postoperative pain: a quantitative systematic review. Pain 81(3):289–297

Ezzo J, Berman B, Hadhazy VA, Jadad AR, Lao L, Singh BB 2000 Is acupuncture effective for the treatment of chronic pain? A systematic review. Pain 86(3):217–225

Johnson MI, Ashton CH, Thompson JW 1992 Long term use of transcutaneous electrical nerve stimulation at Newcastle Pain Relief Clinic. Journal of the Royal Society of Medicine 85(5):267–268

McQuay H, Moore RA 1998 Transcutaneous electrical nerve stimulation (TENS) in chronic pain In: McQuay H, Moore RA (eds) An Evidence-Based Resource for Pain Relief. Oxford University Press, Oxford 207–211

Moher D, Jadad AR, Nichol G, Penman M, Tugwell P, Walsh S 1995 Assessing the quality of randomized controlled trials: an annotated bibliography of scales and checklists. Controlled Clinical Trials 16(1):62–73

Moore A, McQuay H, Gavaghan D 1996 Deriving dichotomous outcome measures from continuous data in randomised controlled trials of analgesics. Pain 66(2-3):229–237

Moore A, Moore O, McQuay H, Gavaghan D 1997 Deriving dichotomous outcome measures from continuous data in randomised controlled trials of analgesics: use of pain intensity and visual analogue scales. Pain 69(3):311–315

Moore A, McQuay H, Gavaghan D 1997 Deriving dichotomous outcome measures from continuous data in randomised controlled trials of analgesics: verification from independent data. Pain 69(1-2):127–130

Moore RA, Gavaghan D, Tramer MR, Collins SL, McQuay H J 1998 Size is everything—large amounts of information are needed to overcome random effects in estimating direction and magnitude of treatment effects. Pain 78(3):209–216

Rundshagen I, Schnabel K, Standl T, Schulte et al 1999 Patients' vs nurses' assessments of postoperative pain and anxiety during patient- or nurse-controlled analgesia. British Journal of Anaesthesia 82(3):374–378

Schulz KF, Chalmers I, Hayes RJ, Altman DG 1995 Empirical evidence of bias. Dimensions of methodological quality associated with estimates of treatment effects in controlled trials. Journal of the American Medical Association 273(5):408–412

Smith LA, Oldman AD, McQuay HJ, Moore RA 2000 Teasing apart quality and validity in systematic reviews: an example from acupuncture trials in chronic neck and back pain. Pain 86(1-2):119–132

Vickers A, Goyal N, Harland R, Rees R 1998 Do certain countries produce only positive results? A systematic review of controlled trials. Controlled Clinical Trials 19(2):159–166

Index

preganglionic neurones (sympathetic system) 29, 30, 32, 33, 40
preganglionic–postganglionic convergence/divergence 32
preganglionic sympathectomy 108
preparing patients for non-medical approaches in low back pain management 182–3, 184
presentation of data 222
prevertebral ganglia 32–3
prostaglandins 95
proximal to distal movement 169
psychophysics 7

questionnaire, low back pain 177–8, 193–200

randomisation 216
randomised controlled trials 215, 216–7, 219, 220
reduction of physiotherapy aids in CRPS patients 169
reflex feedback loops 45–6
reflex sympathetic dystrophy (RSD) see CRPS Type I (RSD)
reliability 212
research evidence, hierarchy of 209
responsiveness 212
risk factors for developing chronic pain 179

sacral parsympathetic outflow 39
saline, role in pain relief 107
'sampling' systems of the CNS 77, 78
and CRPS mechanisms 78
sciatic nerve
chronic constriction injury 112
partial lesions 112
scientific progress, pattern of 6
'scrutinising' systems of the CNS 77
and CRPS mechanisms 84–91
implications for physiotherapists 91–2
sensitisation 85, 87, 88
mind-body link to 88–91
sensory-discriminative, motivational-affective, and central control determinants of pain 10
sensory-immune interaction 97
sensory interaction theory 4, 5
sensory nerve injury, sensitivity states 110

sensory-social restriction, effect on dog's pain perception 7–8
sensory symptoms, CRPS 59
sentient neural hub 13
silent afferents 83
skin conductance, and sympathetic response to physical testing 131–2, 133
slump test 130–1
specificity theory 4, 5, 14
spinal cord, and visceral afferents 45
spinal dorsal horn see dorsal horn
spinal gating mechanism 9
spinal nerve transection model 112
splanchnic nerves 32, 33
splinting in CRPS Type I management 125
stages of CRPS 61–2
statistical tests 222
stellate ganglion 35
stress
and HPA axis activation 48
and increased pain, in CRPS patients 83
and SAM axis activation 48
immune system, and autonomic innervation 47–9
impact on gut 'activity' 41–2
subjective information 212
submucous plexus 41
substance P 65, 85, 95
sudomotor function 131–2
summation theory 4, 5
superior ganglia 32
supersensitivity development, in CRPS 68, 69–70
sympathectomies 108–9, 115
sympathetic adreno-medullary (SAM) axis, and stress 48
sympathetic-afferent coupling 113, 114
sympathetic blocks 105–8
sympathetic ganglia 29
sympathetic nervous system 26–39
and gut 42
and inflammation inhibition 95–6
and manual therapy 127–8, 130–4
clinical implications 35–7
'coupled' to sensory system 93, 96
emotional and cognitive influences 26
in the arm 29
in the lower limbs 30

Review:Topical Issues in Pain 1: Whiplash Science and Management. Fear Avoidance Beliefs and Behaviour. Editor Louis Gifford

By Professor Patrick Wall, best known for the Gate control theory of pain and author of the best selling books 'The Challenge of Pain' (with Ronald Melzack),'Pain the Science of Suffering' and 'The Textbook of Pain' (with Ronald Melzack).

It is not an exaggeration to say that this book marks a milestone not only for an understanding of pain but also for the maturation of physiotherapy. For centuries physiotherapy has been placed in a minor subservient role among the medical arts. This low status encouraged a passive intuitive acceptance of therapy in a barren desert of intellectual questioning. The present rapid evolution of attitude no longer permits untested acceptance. The authors of this book and the organisers of the Physiotherapy Pain Association are clearly pioneers leading their profession out of the desert. They have been reading and experiencing and questioning everything to the conditions, which are treated rather than restricting themselves to the classical physiotherapy texts, which are often dull, repetitive and trivial. In addition to an open-minded education, they point to the almost unique opportunity characteristic of physiotherapy, which remains the close prolonged interaction with patients. Social pressure has removed this from almost every other branch of the medical arts.

The practical pragmatic obsession of old-school physiotherapy assigned questioning and investigation to a separate and distant other class who in practise in fact ignored the problems. Research was assigned to some non-existent class of intellectuals and thought to be beyond the scope of physiotherapists. A striking example is that to be found on page 94 where 20 therapies for whiplash are listed. Of these two are thought to be useless, two useful and the other 16 have not been adequately investigated. This vagueness is a threat to patients and to physiotherapists and to an understanding of pain. Research can not be the responsibility of others. It does not require huge high tech resources. The results are not to be feared. The discovery that a therapy depends on a placebo response should be welcomed with relief because it liberates the therapist into a positive area to explore the economics and the precise nature of the placebo component of the therapy.

Work over the past thirty years has rejected the model of a pain mechanism as caused by a fixed rigid modality-dedicated mechanism. The process, which produces pain, is plastic and changes sequentially with time. That essential mobility of mechanism exists in damaged tissue, in the peripheral nerves and spinal cord. This movement of pathology from periphery to centre proceeds with the triggering of reactive processes in the brain. It presents the therapist with a migrating distributed target. For that reason, I was particularly impressed by the chapter by Gifford on the "Mature Organism Model" which places pain in an integrated context without any permission to accept the old dualistic split that pain must be either in the body or in the mind.

I look forward to this series and to the activities of the Physiotherapy Pain Association because they promise to revolutionise the morale, dignity and way of thinking of physiotherapists and thereby to affect everyone concerned with pain.

Patrick Wall   26.11.98

(Reproduced with permission from : Physiotherapy, February 1999/vol 85/no 2 page 101-102).

Review: Topical Issues in Pain 2: Biopsychosocial assessment and management; Relationships and pain Editor: Louis Gifford

By Gordon Waddell, Consultant Orthopaedic Surgeon and author of 'The Back Pain Revolution'.

The first year book from the Physiotherapy Pain Association was a hard act to follow, but this second year book is even better.

This a diverse collection of essays on selected aspects of pain which is inevitably somewhat disjointed and variable in style and quality, but that lets it explore a number of rarely visited, fascinating topics. Although the authors come from a range of professional backgrounds, they all have considerable "hands on" clinical experience of physiotherapy for patients with pain. Indeed, one of the major achievements and attractions of this book is the highly successful blend of the latest concepts and research on pain with practical illustrations of how that can be applied in practice. That practice ranges all the way from routine out-patient physiotherapy to a tertiary pain management clinic, and the one general criticism is that sometimes the setting of a particular essay is not made clear. For example, lessons from the highly selected patients in a pain management programme are not always applied to more routine practice. However, once the reader realises that different authors may sometimes be talking about different patients, it is possible to draw these lessons from oneself.

Altogether, this is a rich kaleidoscope of the latest thinking and research, which includes some real gems. Each reader will find their own favourites, but a very personal selection that tickled my fancy included the chapters on interpreting the results of treatment, the challenge of change in practice, the impact of patient preferences on treatment outcome, applying yellow flags in clinical practice, pain perceptions and attitudes, and most of the section on "relationships" including in particular pain stories, pain couples and the INPUT Patient Handout on Chronic Pain and Pregnancy. These include some original, highly pertinent and stimulating perspectives. The major achievement and value throughout the book are the many examples of how biopsychosocial principles can be applied in clinical practice.

This is a delightful little book for all physiotherapists and indeed all other health professionals who actually treat patients with pain, not only for those working in pain clinics. The Physiotherapy Pain Association and the editor, Louis Gifford, are once again to be congratulated on producing such a marvellous collection of essays.

Gordon Waddell DSc MD FRCS
(Reproduced with permission Physiotherapy Dec 2000 vol 86(12):665)

Topical Issues in Pain 1

Reader's comments:

'one of the best and most useful Physiotherapy books I've read'

'clinically relevant and up to date stuff'

'keep this sort of material coming!'

Topical Issues in Pain 2

Reader's comments:

'Excellent, another useful and extremely usable book'

'We have found the case history in chapter 4 invaluable in our in-service training of the biopsychosocial model and assessment'

'Should be a standard text in all Physiotherapy undergraduate and post graduate education programmes'

'Easy to read, easy to understand and I've read it from cover to cover (I don't normally get passed chapter 1!!)'.

Topical Issues in Pain 3

Reader's comments:

*'congratulations on Topical Issues in Pain 3,
a tremendous piece of work.'*

'a vital resource'

*'I learnt some more very interesting things about the
sympathetic nervous system, a really comprehensive guide.'*

'the usual high standard and easy to read'

Now Available...

Editor: Louis Gifford

Topical Issues in Pain 1

Introductory Essay	Integrating pain awareness into physiotherapy wise action for the future *David Butler*

Part 1   **Whiplash: science and management**
Michael Thacker, Louis Gifford, Vicki Harding, Suzanne Shorland and Katharine Treves.

Part 2   **Fear avoidance beliefs and behaviour**
Patrick Hill, Dr Michael Rose, Vicki Harding and Max Zusman

Topical Issues in Pain 2

Introductory Essays	The patient in front of us: from genes to environment *Louis Gifford*
	Interpreting the results of treatment *George Peat*

The challenge of change in practice *Heather Muncey*

Exercise for low back pain: clinical outcomes, costs and preferences *Jennifer Klaber Moffett et al.*

Part 1   **Biopsychosocial assessment and management**
Lisa Roberts, Paul Watson, Nicholas Kendall, Jennifer Klaber Moffett

Part 2   **Relationships and pain**
Hazel O'Dowd, Toby Newton-John, Suzanne Brook, Christina Papadopoulos and Vicki Harding

Topical Issues in Pain 3

Introductory Essay	Gate Control Theory – On the Evolution of Pain Concepts, *Ronald Melzack.*

Part 1   **Sympathetic nervous system and pain**
Louis Gifford, Mick Thacker and Suzanne Brook

Part 2   **Pain management**
Chris Main and Paul Watson

Part 3   **Clinical Effectiveness**
Ralph Hammond and Lesley Smith

Topical Issues in Pain 4

Introductory Essay	Introduction to the 4th Edition *Patrick Wall*

Part 1   **Placebo and nocebo**
Patricia Roche, Nigel Lawes, Mitch Noon, Richard Shortall, Caroline Hafner and Louis Gifford

Part 2   **Pain management**
Heather Muncey and Babs Harper

Part 3   **Muscles and pain**
Paul Watson, Patricia Dolan, Lorraine Moores and Ann Papageorgiou